As the founder and director of Australian beauty and wellness brand The Beauty Chef, Carla Oates is a pioneer of the inner beauty industry. She recognised the power of the gut–skin connection while remedying her and her family's skin and health issues. Having worked as a newspaper columnist, beauty editor and stylist, Carla has always been a passionate naturalist and gut-health advocate. She is the author of *Feeding Your Skin* and *The Beauty Chef Cookbook* and has worked as the natural beauty columnist for *WellBeing* magazine for fifteen years. Carla is also an ambassador for Australian Organic. She has been writing, researching and educating her customers about the connection between gut health and beauty and wellbeing for more than a decade. Now, with her third book, Carla explores her philosophy that beauty begins in the belly in new detail.

For Jeet, Otis and Davor, thank you for your love and support
(and patience when I write books), always.

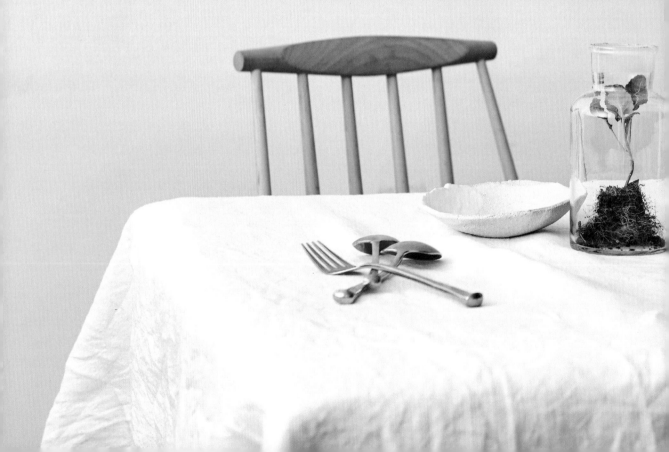

The
Beauty
Chef
Gut
Guide

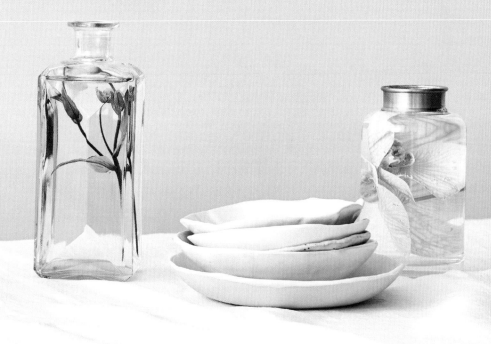

CARLA OATES

Hardie Grant

BOOKS

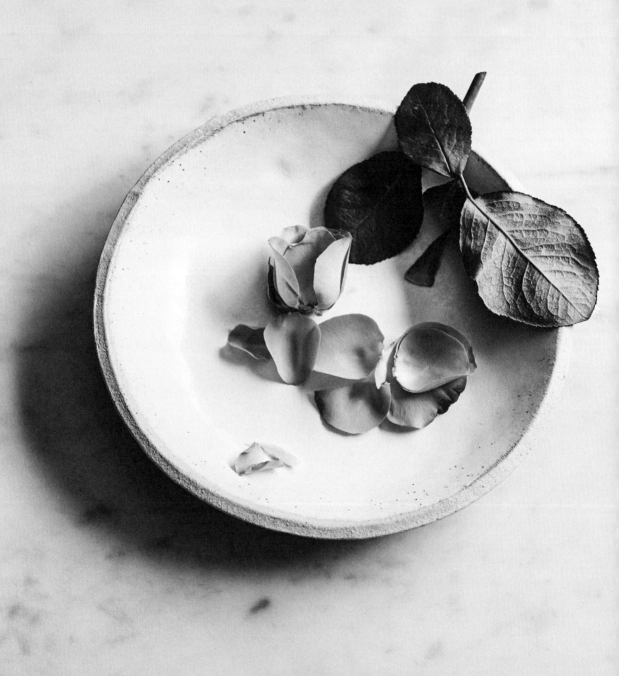

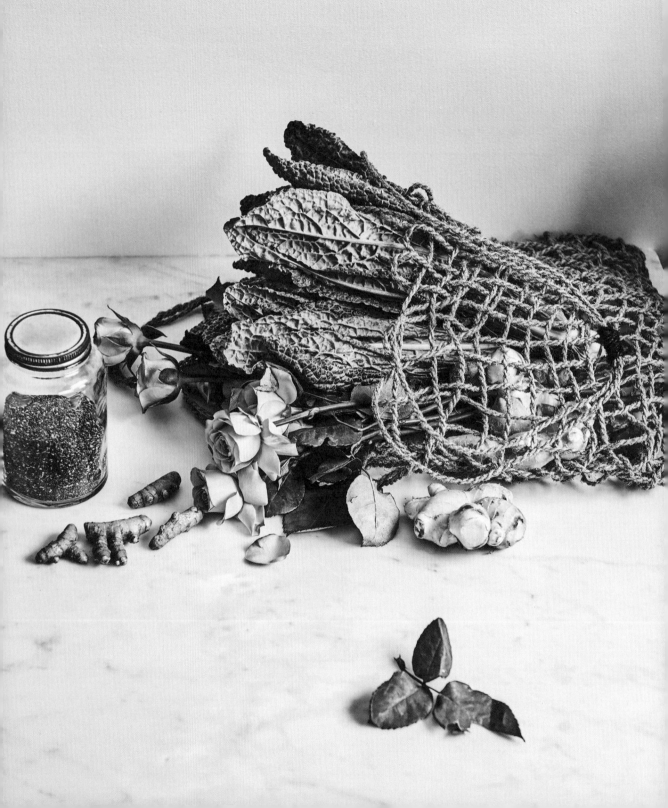

Foreword

by Associate Professor Andrew Holmes

Carla is an enthusiastic advocate for a holistic approach to health and wellbeing that starts with what we eat and how that impacts our gut. Our eating patterns have profound effects on many aspects of our lives that extend well beyond the obvious. In this book, Carla's passion shines through in many ways, and her mission to improve people's health via their gut is one I share. It is a pleasure to have the opportunity to write the foreword for this book.

I am fortunate to be part of the research team at the Charles Perkins Centre at the University of Sydney. Our centre's focus is on finding solutions to three of the major health problems in modern society: obesity, diabetes and cardiovascular disease. All three of these can be described as 'lifestyle diseases', a term that reflects how the epidemiological pattern of these diseases is very strongly associated with our modern lifestyles. As societies have modernised, we have seen increased industrialisation, improved control of infectious diseases, food security and altered work patterns. This has undoubtedly been a good thing for many people, but it has also come with changing disease patterns. We have traded in malnutrition and infectious diseases for 'overnutrition' and chronic non-communicable disease.

The epidemiology of lifestyle diseases does not reflect changes in our genomes or the emergence of new pathogens. Rather, their increased incidence is essentially driven by changes in our environment. This makes understanding these health issues in large part a question of ecology and, particularly, how the availability of food in our environment shapes the human system.

I am interested in our nutritional ecology because I am a microbial ecologist, and humans are symbionts, just like corals. Our body is comprised of trillions of human cells and trillions of microbial cells. When corals are exposed to environmental stresses, such as high nutrient loads in the water, the symbiosis breaks up and coral bleaching results. When humans are exposed to an imbalanced nutrient environment, it too impacts the performance of our symbiosis and our health can suffer. The classic television marketing view of an imbalance between 'good' and 'bad' bugs is an oversimplification, but does have one useful message: what we eat shapes the type of relationship we have with our symbiotic partners.

The relationship between diet, gut microbes and health is strong. It is also important to recognise that it is a complex network. Recognition of this complexity is leading to a revolution in nutrition, whereby old ideas of looking at one nutrient at a time ('Is fat good or bad? Is sugar good or bad?') are being discarded in favour of a holistic approach. A health-promoting diet is not one that glorifies a single 'superfood' or demonises a 'bad food'. It is one that sustains the nutrient needs of your whole body system, including your gut microbes.

So how do we support our gut? An old dictum in microbial ecology is that 'everything is everywhere, but the environment selects'. An even older piece of folk wisdom is, 'You are what you eat'. The majority of us are surrounded by microbes with the potential to develop into either a healthy gut microbial symbiosis or an unhealthy one. How you choose to feed them has arguably the single largest impact on which type of symbiosis develops.

Carla's book offers a comprehensive exploration of gut health and why it matters, including a beautifully presented guide full of recipes that put the food focus where it should be: on creating a happy balance between human and microbe, without sacrificing the enjoyment you get out of your meals.

Associate Professor Andrew Holmes
Charles Perkins Centre at the University of Sydney

Beauty Begins In The Belly

I've always believed that beauty is an inside-out process and that what we eat can have a profound impact on how we look and feel. But this belief is not simply a gut feeling – it stems from my own experience with gut issues.

As a child, I suffered from eczema and allergies. It was only after working with a naturopath, and dramatically changing my diet, that I began to understand the close link between what we eat and our overall health. When my daughter experienced similar health issues, I became even more fascinated by the intimate link between what we eat and the state of our health. Eliminating foods that put stress on our digestive system and introducing fermented foods into my family's diet had a profound impact on not only our skin, but our overall wellbeing. It's this passion for nutrition and fermented foods that has inspired the philosophy at the centre of my brand, The Beauty Chef.

In my book *The Beauty Chef: Delicious Food for Radiant Skin, Gut Health and Wellbeing*, I wanted to bring my story and the evolution of that brand to life – celebrating delicious food and recipes I love to cook and that are beneficial for gut health. With this book, I want to delve a little deeper, examining our relationship with our microbiome. But the premise is the same: food is medicine.

Over the years, I have become even more passionate about the science of food, gut health and the microbiome. With friends, family, colleagues and customers suffering a range of skin and health issues, I am intrigued by how the gut seems to always play a part, influenced greatly by the community of microbes that live there. Problems with gut health and associated diseases are on the rise, and more and more research points to the lack of microbial harmony in our modern-day diets and lifestyles.

It makes sense that the gut has a profound impact on us, considering the intestinal tract contains more chemical detection and signalling molecules than any other organ in the body. What influences gut health above anything else is the community of bugs that reside there and how they behave … or don't.

The question I get asked a lot is: what should we feed our microbes for them to be content and prosper? How do we become a good host to our 'other half'?

I created this book to help people understand, get to know and heal their gut. If your gut is really imbalanced, abruptly changing your diet to foods that should be healthy for you may actually make you feel worse. This is probably because your gut is very much out of balance, in which case these stimulating foods can cause too much action and reaction in the gut. So the first step is to go back to basics, strengthen your gut wall and slowly introduce these healthful foods, which eventually you can eat plentifully – keeping both you, your immune system and your microbes happy.

I am a foodie at heart and have tried to make these recipes as delicious as possible. You will find a diverse range to suit all diets, from morning tonics and tasty lunches to sweet, healthy treats. I don't want you to ever feel like you are depriving yourself, but rather nourishing and nurturing your body.

It is important to love your microbiome: feed, support and embrace it, understanding that it is probably the most significant relationship you will ever have. I wish everyone good gut health, and therefore health and happiness, and hope this book helps you be the best version of you!

Enjoy,
Carla xx

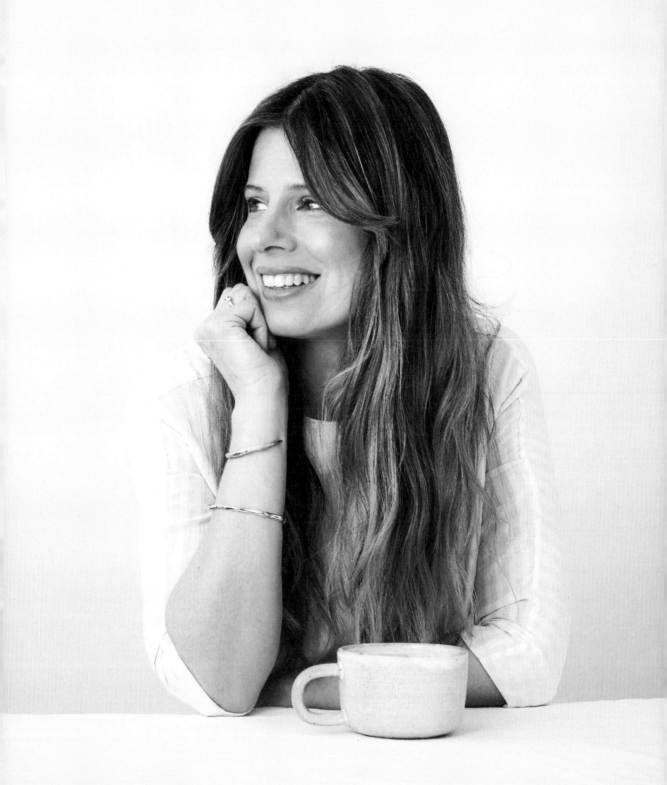

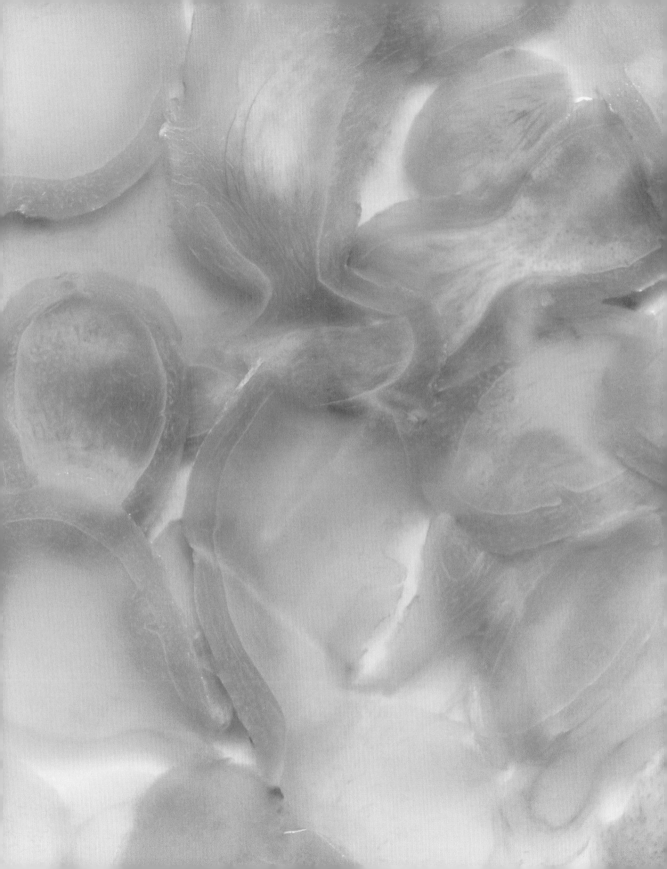

Part 1

Understanding The Gut

Why Your Gut Matters

When you think of the gut, does your mind go straight to your belly? The truth is that our gut, or gastrointestinal tract, runs from our mouths to our derrière and is the gatekeeper to our overall health and immunity. Like our skin, our gut is in constant contact with our external environment, and every day it is faced with a multitude of challenges.

My philosophy has always been that 'beauty begins in the belly' – and it influences everything we do at The Beauty Chef. I truly believe in the power of food as medicine, so it's been wonderful to witness, over the last few years, the building pile of research that supports this philosophy. Every day, more and more studies are shining a light on the intimate link between what we eat, the state of our gut, and our overall health and wellbeing.

At the centre of this research is the gut microbiome. This mini-ecosystem is home to the trillions of microorganisms that populate our digestive tract. Though it's only visible under a microscope, our microbiome, when fully developed, can weigh up to two kilograms! In essence, we have more DNA from bacterial cells than from human cells – our gut is a big part of who we are.

While one of the main roles of the microbiome is to process the food we eat, aiding digestion and assisting in the absorption and synthesis of nutrients, the influence it can have on our health extends far beyond the gut wall. Our microbiota control so much when it comes to health and wellbeing: the mechanics of digestion and metabolising of indigestible compounds, the absorption and assimilation of nutrients, and the manufacture of some vitamins, essential amino acids and bioactive molecules that support our metabolic and immune health, brain function, skin health and mood.

Our gut is like a garden. When healthy, it is full of a diverse range of bacteria that live in symbiosis with the plants that grow within its soil. When it is in balance, or eubiosis, we have a much better chance of experiencing optimal health and wellbeing. But when there is an imbalance, or dysbiosis, we can experience ailments that run the gamut from bloating, fatigue and reflux to headaches, mental health disorders, allergies, and autoimmune and skin conditions.

Many of these health and skin issues are caused by inflammation, which is our body's protective immune response to a perceived threat or injury. Bacterial-derived lipopolysaccharides (LPS), a type of endotoxin, are part of the cell wall of a bacteria type known as Gram negative bacteria. When our gut lining is damaged, these LPS, among other compounds, such as food antigens, can pass through the gut lining (a condition known as leaky gut) into the bloodstream, leading to low-grade systemic inflammation, which is closely linked to many skin and other health conditions. This is why it is important to eat a diet that supports microbial health and, therefore, gut wall integrity.

While acute inflammation – for example, a bruised knee – heals fairly quickly, ongoing or chronic inflammation can be far more problematic. If you have chronic skin inflammation, it is likely you have low-grade gut inflammation as well.

The good news is that our gut health, and overall health, can be improved by being a good host – nurturing our relationship with our microbiome through our diet and lifestyle choices. By strengthening our gut lining and ensuring that we have a good balance of bacteria, our dynamic internal ecosystem can thrive and we can experience good health, vitality and glowing skin. Over the years, this has been one of the greatest pleasures of my job – watching customers nourish their gut health and experience radiant, glowing skin as well as improved health and wellbeing.

Learning how to be a good host, and finding your way to eubiosis, is very empowering.

What Is The Gut?

More than 2000 years ago, Hippocrates – the Greek physician widely referred to as the father of modern medicine – said, 'All disease begins in the gut.' While certainly wise words, scientists have only recently begun to comprehend the truth behind this sentiment.

The gut is one of the most complex systems in the body, home to around 1000 species of bacteria. It consists of living organisms, immune and nervous system cells and hormonal glands. It's where we produce and regulate many essential hormones and neurotransmitters, metabolise nutrients and neutralise pathogens, and where you'll find at least 70 per cent of our immune system.

A CLOSER LOOK AT THE DIGESTIVE SYSTEM

To understand how a malfunctioning gut can lead to disease, it's important to learn what it is and how it works.

THE GUT-BRAIN AXIS

Have you ever been told to 'listen to your gut instinct' or follow a 'gut feeling'? Well, our gut is commonly referred to as our second brain. On a physical level, our gut is influenced by two key systems: the central nervous system (the brain and spinal cord) and the enteric nervous system (located in the gastrointestinal tract), which communicate with one another via the vagus nerve. This information highway is known as the gut–brain axis. The gut is one of your brain's closest confidants and advisers. It produces mood hormones, as well as the hormones cholecystokinin, gastrin, secretin and ghrelin, which convey messages around food and digestion to your brain. These hormonal messages help regulate appetite, digestion, energy and blood sugar levels.

THE 'YUM' CONNECTION

Have you ever wondered why a plate of food can get you salivating before you've had a single bite? The initial stage of digestion, called the cephalic phase (in Latin, *ceph* means 'head'), can be triggered by the mere thought, emotion or memory of food, as well as its smell, sight and taste. These sensory stimuli activate the brain, which sends signals down the vagus nerve to the gut. Salivating kickstarts the secretion of digestive juices in the stomach, which is our body's way of preparing for the arrival of food and later assists in the digestion, transportation and utilisation of key nutrients. The old saying 'we eat with our eyes' is true, and just one reason why taking the time to prepare a delicious, nutrient-dense meal is so important. I'm far more likely to enjoy a meal if it looks as delicious and nourishing as possible.

THE MOUTH

Your mum was right to tell you to chew your food properly! Mechanical and chemical digestion begins in the mouth. Chewing each mouthful until it's almost liquid helps the food mix in with salivary and digestive enzymes. This kicks off the chemical digestion of carbohydrates and fats and sends signals to the rest of the gut that food is on its way. In response, digestive glands secrete mucus, acids, juices and enzymes into the gut in preparation.

THE STOMACH

When food reaches our stomach in the upper abdomen, digestive juices and acids are released. Waves of contractions churn the food over the course of several hours, mixing it with these acidic juices to break down its chemical bonds into a semi-fluid mass called chyme. This is then pumped into the small intestine for the next stage of processing.

THE SMALL INTESTINE

Despite its name, this intestine is the longest and hardest-working section of the digestive tract, measuring roughly three to four times the body's height. It's where digestion really kicks into gear. You know that feeling when your stomach rumbles? It's actually your small intestine, and you can only hear the sound so clearly because your digestive tract is clear.

Chyme enters it from the stomach, where it's mulched up much the same way garden soil is churned by repeated tilling. Digestive enzymes such as lipase, protease and amylase are released from the pancreas and the gut wall, further breaking down proteins, carbohydrates and fats. Some of the nutrients from the chyme are transported through the gut wall into the surrounding blood vessels and are taken to the liver for processing.

The wall of the small intestine is covered in absorptive villi (tiny finger-like hairs), which enhance and optimise the absorption and transportation of nutrients. They are made up of epithelial cells, which are covered in microvilli (often referred to as a brush border). These are crucial for digestion – fixed to their surface is an abundance of essential digestive enzymes. Together, these villi and microvilli create a surface area that's 600 times greater than if the small intestine were a simple smooth tube.

When the villi are damaged or irritated, digestion and absorption of key nutrients can be impaired. The good news is that the intestinal epithelium (intestinal lining) is thought to regenerate every five to seven days. While it's constantly battered – subjected to the wear and tear that comes with digesting and transporting food, breaking down and absorbing nutrients, and processing toxins and waste – it's also incredibly resilient.

THE LARGE INTESTINE

The next stop is the large intestine: the two-metre-long tube that houses the largest proportion of our microbes. This is where we want them to be, fermenting fibre and producing gut-loving, anti-inflammatory compounds called short-chain fatty acids (page 40). Chyme enters at the caecum, just above the appendix, and slowly moves towards the rectum, ready for excretion. Gentle waves of contractions from the intestinal wall help to move things along. If things are working well, the result is a healthy bowel motion the shape and consistency of a ripe banana.

BUILDING YOUR BACTERIAL BLUEPRINT

The human body is host to around 100 trillion microbes. You'll find them everywhere – on our skin, in our hair and in our mouth – but our gut is home to the largest proportion of them. Before we are born, we are entirely free of microbes; our gut is a blank canvas, and it takes around three years for us to develop our own unique bacterial blueprint. Our microbiome is entirely unique to us, just like our fingerprints. No two are quite alike.

The development of this blueprint starts at birth. Whether we're delivered vaginally or by Caesarean section plays an important role in the development of our microbiome. When babies are born vaginally, they are rapidly colonised by their mum's bacteria while passing through the birth canal. That is one reason why a mum's gut health is important during pregnancy, as healthy (and unhealthy) bugs are passed to the baby during birth.

The rest of our microbial composition comes down to the microorganisms we come into contact with once we're out in the world: in the hospital, while being passed around to friends and family members for cuddles, arriving at home to be licked by the dog and, of course, through breastfeeding. For babies delivered by Caesarean, breastfeeding may be even more important, since the hospital environment is the first thing they come into contact with. While research is ongoing, some studies[1] suggest that early disruption to the gut microbiota may lead to allergies like asthma, eczema and even obesity in later life. While your mode of birth may influence whether or not the immune system is primed to be susceptible to allergic disorders, what we consume post-birth also impacts our microbiome. Breastfeeding is bifidogenic; in other words, it promotes the growth of beneficial bacteria in the intestinal tract, including *Bifidobacteria*. Breast milk also contains antibodies, which help to bolster a baby's immune system and support their ongoing health.

It's important to remember that the relationship we have with our microbiome is a mutual one. We, the host, provide microbes with nutrients and a homely, stable environment – a healthy garden in which to grow. Although our microbial blueprint is pretty well-developed and 'set' by the age of three, our inner ecosystem and relationship with our microbiome are constantly evolving and change as we age. We can positively affect our bacterial composition through our diet and lifestyle choices – in as little as a day.

BEYOND 'GOOD' & 'BAD' MICROBIOTA

While it makes sense to want to separate microbes into two distinct categories – good and bad – it's just not that simple. There are well over 150 different phyla, or groups, of microorganisms, in our bodies. In our gut, the bacteria predominantly belong to two major phyla, Bacteroidetes and Firmicutes, but that's only scratching the surface.

The incredible number and diversity of bacterial species in our gut is hard to comprehend, so in some ways it's easier to think about them like this: there are microbes that we want (fibre degraders) and ones we don't (pathogens), but the truth is that there are types that can be good and bad, or relatively neutral, depending on the microbes' interactions within their environment.

BACTERIA & THEIR IMPACT

1   *Bacteria we always want.* These are species and strains of bacteria that generally serve us well. These 'good' guys work with us in a number of ways, helping with nutrient absorption, detoxification, and in supporting immune function and neurotransmitter production.

2   *Bacteria we want, but only in the right way.* Some bacteria can exhibit both helpful and harmful behaviours. For example, some produce pro-inflammatory compounds which, when we're young, help train our immune systems. These same compounds can be harmful later in life if they create an imbalance in our microbiome.

3   *Bacteria we don't want.* Also known as pathogenic bacteria, their presence can result in digestive symptoms such as bloating, indigestion, abdominal pain, frequent or loose bowel motions, or constipation.

While we don't want pathogenic bacteria, our aim is to strike a healthy balance between the different types of bacteria in our gut – and for them to live together harmoniously with us, their host. In fact, more than 95 per cent of bacteria are harmless to us. It's only when a bacterial imbalance occurs that our skin and health suffer. And while we want 'beneficial' bacteria, it's important to remember that they can behave badly in certain contexts – namely, if our gut health is not in balance, or if we are suffering from leaky gut (page 23). This is why healing the gut is essential for microbial balance.

Are You A Good Host?

In any relationship, when one party is out of balance it can throw the other one into a state of instability. Dysbiosis occurs when there is an imbalance between us, the human (host) system, and our microbiome. When we are stressed, it is likely our microbiome is too.

What we eat determines the fate of our microbes. It's not just about the types of food we eat, but our pattern of consumption – how many meals a day, the size of the meal and its composition.

Our relationship with our gut is always evolving. I'm sensitive to gluten and dairy, so these are two things I removed from my diet. When I did, I noticed a significant improvement in my allergies and eczema. But now, after years of nourishing my body with nutrient-dense wholefoods and probiotic-rich fermented foods, I find that I can indulge every now and then without detrimental side effects. If I overindulge, however (which can happen now and then, especially if I'm travelling), or if I feel stressed, my skin is one of the first places to show symptoms of a gut imbalance.

Microbiologist Dr Andrew Holmes says that fostering a healthy relationship with your microbiome is all about understanding that we are a holobiont: an organism composed of multiple partners living in symbiosis. The general principle is 'eat to share'. Different bacteria feed on different nutrients, so you want to eat a healthy, balanced diet that covers all nutrient groups.

GUIDELINES FOR EATING TO SHARE

- Eat enough to meet the demands of all partners in the holobiont: your body and your microbiome.

- Having more than what you need is not good. Don't eat more than either partner needs, as that creates an unbalanced partnership.

- Eat in a way that allows all partners the time and space to get what they need: eat nutrient-balanced foods in a regular pattern that includes rest periods.

- Recognise and use the different strengths of each partner – fibre plays to the strengths of your microbiome.

- What your microbiome needs is not necessarily the same as your friend's microbiome. We are all individuals, so respect the boundaries and needs of your own system.

- The most important thing your microbiome needs is what it has least of. Look at your diet and lifestyle to figure out what it's missing.

- Eat more fibre and less meat, while always keeping balance and diversity in mind.

BALANCE IS KEY

Both protein and fat are considered essential nutrients for growth, reproductive health, healthy hormones, neurotransmitters and gut health, so it's important to maintain a balanced diet no matter your food philosophy. We should take the same attitude to our diet as we do to our bacteria – everything in balance. There's no reason to cut out meat if you're looking to improve your gut health. Simply eat it in moderation and enjoy it alongside fibre-rich plant foods. Fibre works in favour of your immune and metabolic health, but you still need to eat enough protein for your basic biological needs. As Dr Holmes says, 'As a general rule, everything in nutrition is about balance. Avoiding meat simply creates a different kind of imbalance to having too much meat. A healthy diet balances a moderate amount of meat with good sources of complex carbohydrates, fibre and phytochemicals.'

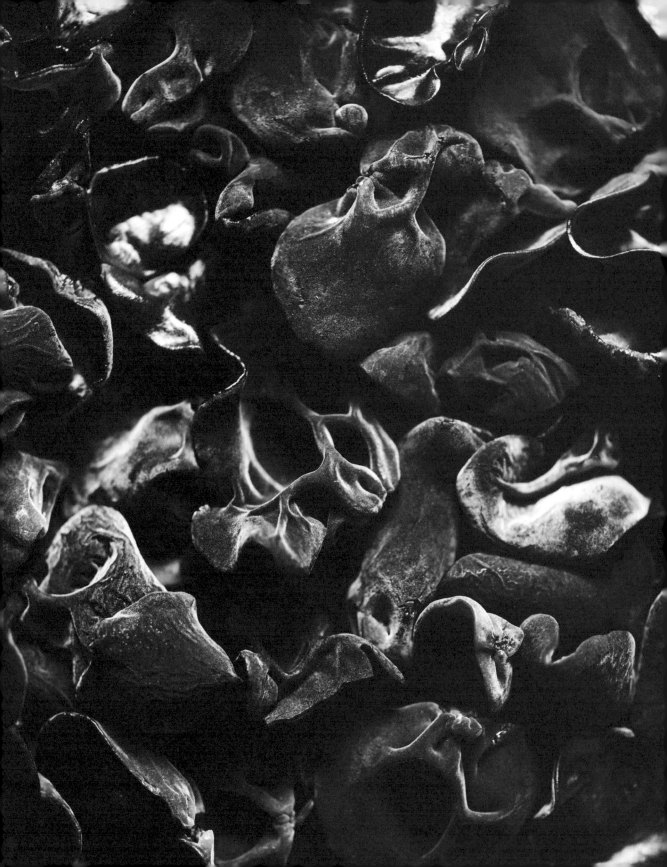

Factors That Compromise Your Gut Health

A number of factors can damage the gut's delicate lining, letting LPS, a type of endotoxin (which are a part of the cell wall of Gram negative bacteria, rather than the whole bacterium), pass through the gut wall and into the bloodstream. Understanding what these factors are, and how to avoid or mitigate them, will set you on the road to optimal gut health – and give you the knowledge you need to recognise when something's not quite right.

HARMFUL FOODS

What we choose to eat can either help to heal our gut or harm it. Consuming refined sugars, preservatives, refined flours, additives, MSG, alcohol, and charred or burnt food can all contribute to dysbiosis, toxin overload and inflammation, which damages the delicate epithelial cells and microvilli of the gut wall. Some research shows that gluten may be particularly harmful and pose issues for some people (page 36). One study shows that gliadin[2], a protein found in wheat, actually increases intestinal permeability and leaky gut (page 23) whether you're gluten-sensitive, coeliac or not. If you're battling with gut issues, it's worth removing gluten from your diet to see if it's the culprit.

Any hard-to-digest molecule can potentially trigger an immune response. For some, dairy, corn and soy produce similar symptoms to gluten sensitivities, and protein – whether from animal foods or unfermented dairy – can also be difficult to break down, especially for those with impaired gut health. If you're experiencing gut issues that get worse after eating certain foods, you want to simplify your diet so you can identify your triggers (page 59).

FOOD PRODUCTION

Though our world is 'cleaner' than ever, an overload of chemical toxins and our obsession with hygiene have had a huge impact on the microbial world. Pesticides, herbicides and genetically modified foods are all too common, and there simply isn't enough evidence to show that they are safe for us to consume over the long term. With the growth of mass agriculture and monoculture, soils are becoming nutrient poor. Minerals such as zinc, selenium and iodine are less prevalent in our soil, yet they are critical to our gut health.

Supporting sustainable agriculture and opting for organically grown or biodynamic produce is therefore key. By doing so, you're helping to rebuild healthy, nutrient-rich soils, which leads to better produce, healthier people and a happier planet. It's sometimes hard to get to the farmers' market, so why not join a local organic co-op or create your own within your local community – you can buy organic fare in bulk and divvy it up among friends and neighbours.

MEDICATION & ANTIBIOTICS

While there's no question that the advent of antibiotics has saved countless lives and given us tools to treat a myriad of bacterial infections, they may also harbour negative side effects. Research shows that even a single course of antibiotics may forever alter the bacterial profile of our gut[3]. The medicinal purpose of antibiotics is to eliminate the pathogens that are making us sick. The trouble is that some don't discriminate between different kinds of bacteria, wiping out everything in their path. They can also potentially reduce our gut's microbial diversity, which is essential for optimal health and wellbeing. Other medications, such as oral contraceptive pills and non-steroidal anti-inflammatories (such as Aspirin), may have a similar effect.

STRESS

When we're stressed, the stress hormone cortisol is released into our bloodstream. While short bouts of stress are normal and can, in fact, be beneficial when we're faced with a challenge, ongoing or chronic stress can wreak havoc on our wellbeing and our gut. Studies show that stress can alter the balance of bacteria in our gut and damage the gut lining[4]. High levels of cortisol also suppress our immune system, making us increasingly vulnerable to pathogens and infection. This influx of cortisol is bad news for our skin, too, as cortisol breaks down collagen, the protein that keeps our skin strong and plump. Stress and emotional upset lead to skin inflammation and can exacerbate skin conditions such as psoriasis, eczema, acne and rosacea. This is certainly true for me. If I'm stressed, or not taking time to relax and rest, my skin is the first place to show signs of it.

ENVIRONMENTAL TOXINS

To understand how environmental toxins impact gut health, it helps to remember that we are biological beings that have a synergy with our environment. Just as chemicals and toxins stress our planet's ecosystems, they also put strain on our internal one.

No matter how many nutrient-dense foods we consume in an effort to nourish our gut, our busy modern lives and exposure to environmental toxins can still alter the balance and diversity of our gut microbiome. While these toxins are commonly found in our water, cleaning products and personal care products, the good news is that we can reduce our toxic load (page 43) by choosing clean and green products, as well as putting filters on our taps. Everyday mycotoxins, or toxic moulds, such as mould in our homes, and poor air quality, can cause allergies and inflammation. So even if you're not experiencing gut issues, if you suffer from allergies or sinus problems it may be worth investigating your home environment with the aim to detoxify it.

NUTRIENT DEFICIENCIES

Nutrient deficiencies and leaky gut (page 23) can 'cause and effect' one another. Micronutrient deficiencies (such as zinc, vitamin C, selenium, vitamin A and magnesium) and macronutrient deficiencies (amino acids found in protein), as well as a lack of fibre, can contribute to the development of leaky gut, as these nutrients are vital to keeping the gut strong and healthy. If you're suffering from leaky gut you may also be battling with nutrient deficiencies, as the gut is less able to absorb and assimilate key nutrients.

A LITTLE DIRT DOESN'T HURT

A number of interesting studies have examined the link between microbial diversity, allergies and asthma, forming what has been known as the 'hygiene hypothesis', which states that less exposure to bacteria and germs during childhood leads to more allergies in adulthood[5,6]. A 2016 observational study, which looked at 10,000 adults across fourteen countries, revealed that children who had grown up in farm environments – with exposure to a greater diversity of microbes – were 54 per cent less likely to have asthma and hay fever in adulthood compared to those who grew up in urban environments[7].

Understanding The Gut

The most integral factor concerning gut health is the concept of microbial diversity – when it comes to gut microbes, diversity is a very good thing. A diverse microbial community is vital for our health and disease prevention, according to microbiome studies[8].

One of my favourite sayings in microbiology is 'everything is everywhere, but the environment selects'. By 'everything' we mean microbes: beneficial, pathogenic and indifferent bacteria are always there, both in the food we eat and in our environment, and our choices in regards to what we eat and our lifestyle practices will encourage the beneficial or not-so-beneficial bugs that we are exposed to. Humans used to forage for foods rich in microbes and consumed plants and their fibre-rich roots. Our modern-day lifestyle has brought us convenient, processed foods that are low in fibre and often nutritionally imbalanced. Highly processed food promotes much lower diversity and, worse, may feed pathogenic bacteria.

To foster diversity, opt for a nutritionally balanced, diverse diet that includes fibre and plenty of wholefoods to create optimal conditions for different bacteria. Avoid a diet dominated by processed, easy-to-digest foods; if digestion only happens in the small intestine, then you are not providing food for the beneficial bugs in the colon. At the same time, we needn't be so clinical about our attitude to food and its preparation – a little dirt never hurt anyone. Gardening, and exposing ourselves to soil-based organisms, may also help boost our gut's diversity, as can fermented foods (pages 37 & 44).

GEOGRAPHY MATTERS

Believe it or not, geography can have an impact on microbial composition. A 2010 study examined the gut bacteria of European children, comparing them with kids who grew up in rural Africa[9]. The diets of the two groups were quite different: European children consumed more processed, or 'Western', foods compared to the African children's largely plant-based diet. Not surprisingly, the bacteria living in the guts of these children were completely different too. The African children had more types of bacteria overall, many of which possess anti-inflammatory properties – able to combat the harmful inflammation that increases someone's risk of disease. Some of the healthy bacteria living in their bellies weren't found in European children, who simply had fewer types of bacteria. This further emphasises my philosophy that we are better off eating foods that are as natural and close to our environment as possible to give our gut the best possible chance to thrive. Even by taking the small step of growing your own herbs or veggies at home in soil you touch and cultivate yourself, your health – and that of your microbiome – will undoubtedly benefit.

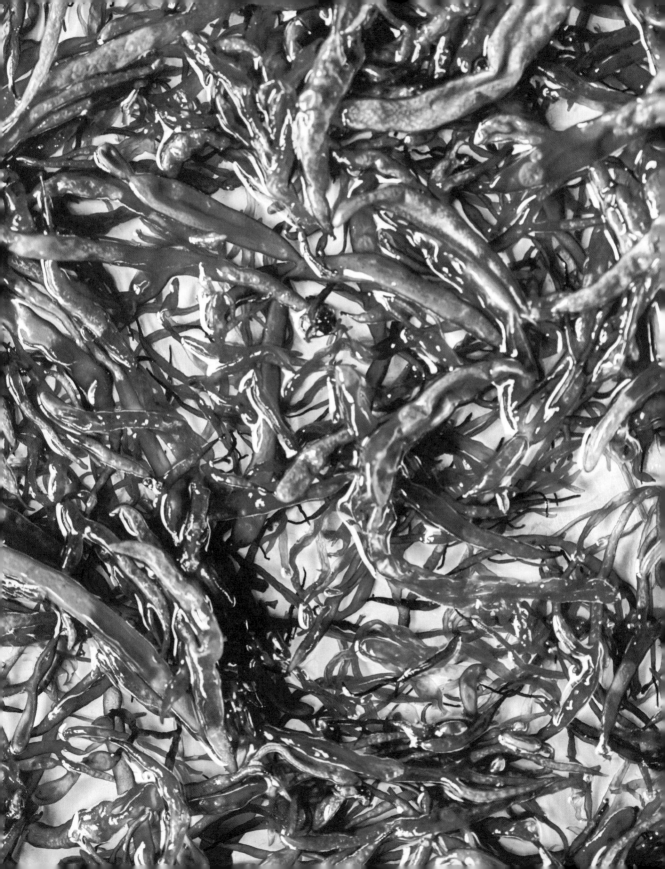

Is Your Symptom Or Health Issue Caused By Your Gut?

It can be difficult to make sense of if, and how, your gut health might be linked to your health condition or discomfort. But considering that the bulk of our immune system is located in the gut, it's no surprise that an imbalance there can trigger a wave of symptoms and health complications. Think of it this way: if the soil in a garden isn't healthy and nutrient balanced, plants aren't able to grow and thrive as they should. The same is true in our gut. An imbalanced, unhealthy gut microbiome leads to low-grade systemic inflammation, which is one of the key drivers for chronic disease. Healing your gut is often the best step you can take towards wellbeing.

When our gut seems to be running smoothly, we don't give it too much thought. But when there's trouble, our body is quick to alert us with a few key signs and symptoms. The secret to keeping our gut happy and healthy lies in learning to read and pay attention to those signs, and to know what to test for and treat when we see them.

LEAKY GUT

Often thought to be an underlying cause of most gut and skin issues, leaky gut syndrome – or intestinal permeability – literally means that the integrity of the gut wall has been compromised, arousing an immune response. In a healthy gut, the mucosal wall forms a barrier between the external environment (the food we eat) and our internal body. The epithelial cells of the gut wall contain tight junctions that allow vital nutrients to be absorbed and assimilated into the body; in a leaky gut, these tightly woven junctions become more permeable than they should be, allowing some compounds from the gut (such as LPS and food antigens, see page 13) to escape into the bloodstream instead of being processed and eliminated. The body responds to these escapees as if they're foreign invaders, which causes inflammation.

The causes of leaky gut can be complex and multi-layered, and include diet, stress, medications, alcohol, parasites and yeast overgrowth, which can damage the epithelial cells and trigger an immune response. If the small intestine is overrun with bacteria (which should reside predominately in the large intestine), it can compromise the protective lining of the gut.

The symptoms of leaky gut vary from person to person and depend on your genetics as well as the state of your gut – your genome as well as your microbiome. Obtaining a clinical diagnosis can also be difficult, as many of the symptoms aren't specific to leaky gut alone. If you suspect you're suffering from leaky gut, it's worth consulting with a skilled naturopath or integrative doctor.

TESTING FOR LEAKY GUT

The simplest way to test for leaky gut is to undergo intestinal permeability screening. This test requires you to drink some lactulose. Its molecules are normally too large to pass through the intestinal epithelium, but if leaky gut is present, it is absorbed across the gut wall and excreted in your urine. Urine is collected over the course of six hours to determine how much of the sugar has been absorbed, which offers insight into whether or not you have leaky gut and how severe it might be.

Common symptoms of leaky gut:

· Bloating

· Burping or flatulence

· Constipation and/or diarrhoea

· Cramping and/or pain in the intestines

· Nausea

MALABSORPTION

The main role of the small intestine is to digest the food we eat and absorb all the goodness and nutrients that we need to thrive. If you're suffering from malabsorption issues, it means your small intestine is having difficulty absorbing nutrients and allowing them to be used effectively. While leaky gut and malabsorption issues are sometimes related, and you can have issues with both, they aren't the same thing. Leaky gut compromises the gut wall, while malabsorption indicates that nutrients aren't being absorbed properly.

Digestive enzymes play a key part in this process, breaking down food into specific nutrient components. Digestive enzymes are produced in the pancreas, small intestine, stomach and salivary glands – without them, our body would be starved of nutrients. Digestive enzymes can help reduce the adverse effects of food intolerances; when food is broken down, there's less chance of endotoxins and allergenic proteins (created by undigested food particles) crossing the gut wall and irritating the immune system. Consistent irritation can actually contribute to ongoing allergies.

While supplementation can certainly be helpful, these clever enzymes are also naturally found in food. Bromelain, found in pineapple, and papain, found in papaya, both help break down proteins. Fermented foods also contain beneficial bacteria species that help with the digestion of some foods[10].

Factors that can compromise the effectiveness of our digestive enzymes:

· Intestinal damage, either through illness, infection or trauma

· Prolonged use of antibiotics

· Leaky gut

· Parasites or yeast or bacterial overgrowth (for example, SIBO or candida, see page 28)

· A poor diet or eating too quickly

· Low levels of stomach acid

DO YOU NEED TO BOOST YOUR DIGESTIVE ENZYMES?

To treat malabsorption, you have to recognise the symptoms, which can differ depending on the nutrient (or nutrients) you are having trouble absorbing.

If you're suffering from one or more of these symptoms, it may be a sign you need to boost your digestive enzymes:

· Indigestion within 1–3 hours of eating

· Oil and/or undigested food in stools

· Smelly or excessive flatulence or foul-smelling stools

· Diagnosed vitamin or mineral deficiencies

· Increasing food intolerances or allergies

· Nausea after eating fats, even if mild

Different enzymes are helpful in breaking down different food components:

· Protease breaks down proteins into amino acids

· Lipase breaks down lipids/fats into fatty acids and glycerol

· Amylase breaks down carbohydrates and starches into sugars

PROTEIN DEFICIENCY

After water, protein is the most plentiful substance found in our body, and it forms the structure of our skin, hair, nails, organs, gut lining, muscles, tendons and ligaments. It also plays a role in the production of hormones and helps our body fight disease. One of our most abundant proteins, collagen, makes up 75 to 80 per cent of the skin's structure. So it's essential that we consume enough protein and that our body is able to break it down. We are able to synthesise non-essential amino acids, but there are nine that our body is unable to produce on its own and that we must get from our diet.

Symptoms that indicate you may have trouble breaking down proteins or don't have enough good-quality ones in your diet:

· Bad breath

· Burping or bloating

· Dry, split or brittle hair

· Food allergies or intolerances

· General malaise or compromised immune function

· Heaviness after a protein-rich meal

· Hormone imbalances or deficiencies

· Loss of skin tone and elasticity or thin, lined, dull skin

· Lymphatic congestion

· Muscle wasting and fat gain

· Poor wound healing

· Reduced liver detoxification

· Foul-smelling flatulence

· Weak or peeling nails, vertical ridges

IMBALANCED DIETARY FAT INTAKE

Research is increasingly showing that our clever gut microbiota regulate the digestion and absorption of dietary fats, but we have to play our part by choosing the right ones[11]. Eating healthy fats is vital for our overall health and wellbeing – fats play an essential role in healthy skin. But it's not just about eating the right types of fat, it's also about ratio. Both omega-6 and omega-3 fatty acids are considered essential. The trouble with our highly processed Western diet is that most of us are eating a ratio that's far out of balance – around 16 to 1 – and too much omega-6 can lead to inflammation. Instead, a ratio of 4 to 1 – four omega-6 to one omega-3 – is recommended (some health experts even suggest a ratio of 1 to 1). We should all be consuming more anti-inflammatory omega-3 fatty acids (found in oily fish, nuts, seeds, eggs, vegetables and grass-fed meat) – omega-3s can increase the number of beneficial bacteria in your gut and promote microbial diversity[12]. To help boost my intake, I often add chia seeds to my smoothie, or sardines and/or walnuts to my lunch salad bowls.

These symptoms may indicate you have issues with fat digestion:

· General heaviness in the gut

· Nausea or headaches after eating fatty foods, especially behind the eyes or at the back of the head

· Pale, fatty, slimy or loose stools

· Dry, flaky, itchy skin, brittle nails or dull hair

· Pain in the gallbladder or mid-back

· Yellow tinge in the whites of the eyes/the skin

CARBOHYDRATE DIGESTION

Specific enzymes are required to break down specific carbohydrates, so an enzyme deficiency is likely to produce unpleasant symptoms. Take a lack of lactase, for example: that's the enzyme required to digest the lactose found in dairy products. Many people discover that by ditching dairy (or at least lactose), they see a significant improvement in their skin. Acne and eczema, in particular, are closely correlated with dairy consumption, as are bloating and diarrhoea.

Blood-sugar imbalances can also be associated with faulty carbohydrate digestion. The glycaemic index (GI) measures how quickly a food releases energy (glucose) into our blood. The higher the food's GI, the quicker and higher blood sugar levels rise, triggering the pancreas to release insulin to shift glucose from the blood into cells to use or store. A rapid rise in blood sugar that occurs regularly due to faulty carbohydrate digestion can spark a surge in insulin, which can manifest as gut and skin problems.

Common symptoms that indicate carbohydrate digestion issues:

· Bloating and flatulence after eating carbohydrate-rich foods

· Blood sugar spikes and energy level crashes after meals

· Having to eat every few hours to avoid extreme hunger, irritability or confusion

· Raised serum fasting insulin levels

· Sugar cravings, particularly after meals

The spectrum of allergies and intolerances is broad, and while we can be genetically predisposed to different immune response pathways, allergies are not necessarily 'hardwired' into our system. A leaky gut (page 23) can create temporary allergies or sensitivities. When the gut is leaky and, therefore, more permeable, molecules that wouldn't normally cross the gut wall barrier can trigger an immune response as our body tries to deal with what it sees as an invader.

But you don't necessarily have to live with allergies and intolerances. What you choose to eat, and how you choose to live, can impact which of our genes are turned 'on' or 'off' at any given time. I experienced this firsthand when I changed my diet to clear up my eczema. It was incredible to see the improvement in just a few weeks.

In our Gut Guide, we eliminate all gluten and dairy from the diet. Wheat contains two inflammatory proteins, gluten and lectins, that research shows may increase gut permeability and inflammation[13]. Gluten may also contribute to brain fog, or mental fuzziness, when these molecules pass into the bloodstream. Some research suggests[14] that the effects of gliadin and glutenin – two components found in gluten – actually act like opioids, causing brain fog and lethargy. Dairy contains lactose and beta-casein, which many people have trouble tolerating[15]. Clinically speaking, removing gluten and dairy is common practice when working to heal the gut. Many practitioners agree that gut function and skin conditions improve much faster by steering clear of these substances for a period of time.

While gluten and dairy are common culprits, if the gut is chronically damaged and an inflammatory immune response has been triggered, your immune system can even react to healthy foods. You may be able to work out yourself what those foods are, but you also may need to work alongside a practitioner on eliminating reactive foods.

After you've completed the Gut Guide, you'll be able to slowly add these foods back into your diet and assess your reaction to them. If there's no adverse response, you may find you can enjoy them occasionally with no harmful effects. If you experience an obvious reaction, then it's wise to remove these substances for another few weeks until you settle the gut again and seek additional advice from your health care practitioner.

HISTAMINE INTOLERANCE

Histamine is a naturally occurring chemical involved with your immune, digestive and central nervous systems that responds to any potential attackers. It is a normal protective response, but if you have trouble breaking down histamine you can develop a histamine intolerance. Leaky gut (page 23) often fuels your histamine intolerance. Our naturopaths and nutritionists have found that once leaky gut is healed and liver function improved, histamine issues usually calm down.

A variety of foods are naturally high in histamines, including fermented foods, shellfish, beans and pulses, smoked meat, walnuts, cacao, pickled foods and matured cheeses.

Symptoms of histamine intolerance include:

· Skin rashes and hives

· Persistent fatigue

· Flushing and sweating

· Dry and tearing eyes

· Scent/chemical reactions

· Temperature sensitivity

Using natural antihistamines regularly, improving gut function and managing stress levels all help to reduce histamine sensitivity. To start with, reduce or avoid high-histamine foods as well as the fermented foods suggested in the Gut Guide if you feel better without them. You can add them slowly at the end of the program when your gut has improved.

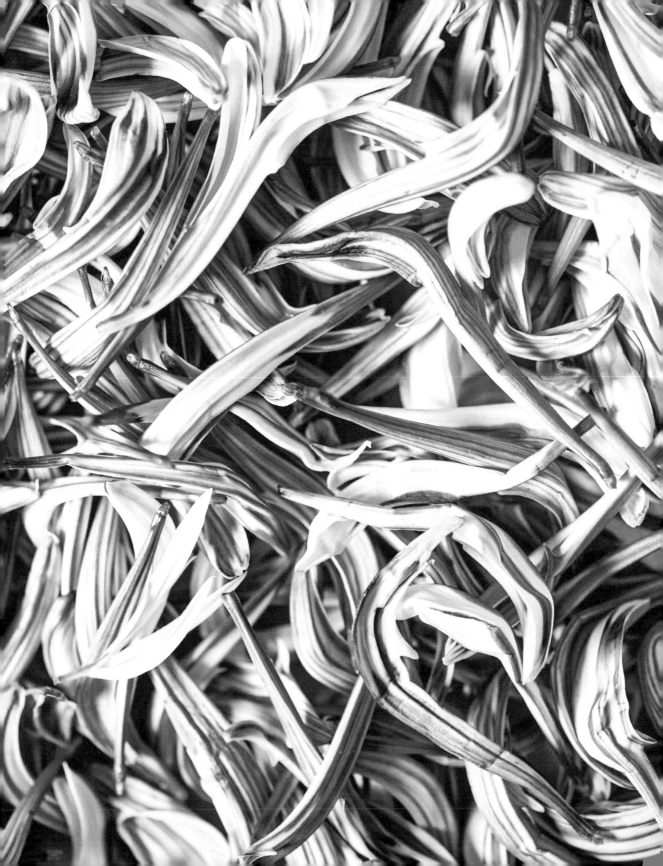

While not technically a gut disorder, sex and stress hormone issues and imbalances can be directly linked to gut health. Cortisol (our stress hormone) can impact our gut health profoundly (see page 20). But digestive health can also impact your oestrogen levels. Similar to the gut–brain axis, there is an oestrogen–gut microbiome axis. Your gut microbiota produce an enzyme called ß-glucuronidase that breaks down oestrogen into its active form. If you have dysbiosis and lower microbial diversity, your gut bugs won't produce enough of this enzyme, which results in less circulating active (useful) oestrogen and more bound (ready for excretion) oestrogen. If your elimination pathways aren't working efficiently, bound oestrogen will be re-circulated, resulting in an imbalance/excess of oestrogen in your body.

Oestrogen influences more than you might think, from fat deposition and obesity through to improving bone health and protecting cardiovascular health[16]. To avoid oestrogen imbalance, it's important to make and eliminate this hormone efficiently by supporting gut and liver health, as well as having a good microbial balance.

An excess of oestrogen can also be caused by xenoestrogens. They are hormone-mimicking compounds that interrupt our endocrine system and wreak havoc on our gut health. Found in every-day items including plastic, make-up and skincare products, and non-organic fruits and vegetables, they are difficult to break down and often get trapped in our system and stored in our fat cells. When they build up in our bodies, it can lead to oestrogen dominance and symptoms like adrenal fatigue[17], bloatedness, mood swings, fluid retention, acne and breast tenderness, to name but a few. Hence, we need to make sure that our body has access to our naturally occurring oestrogens and doesn't look to use xenoestrogens, which is why it's important to keep our microbes happy and our excretion pathways working properly.

SIBO is a bacterial overgrowth in the small intestine that creates greater competition between us and our microbes for essential nutrients. Most of our gut bacteria are located in the large intestine (or colon), so when the small intestine is overrun we can experience myriad symptoms and issues: malabsorption, bloating, diarrhoea and nutrient deficiencies, as well as damage to the gut wall and an increased risk of developing leaky gut (see page 23). If you have diminished gastric acid secretion, small intestine dysmotility and disruptions in gut immune function, you'll probably have to contend with bacterial overgrowth.

If you suspect you have SIBO, pay attention to the following signs:

· Bloating

· Nausea

· Skin issues including rashes, acne, eczema or rosacea

· Joint pain

· Mood issues or depression

· Diarrhoea

CANDIDA

Candida albicans is a yeast that isn't a problem for everyone, but an overgrowth – often caused by poor diet, medications and compromised gut and immune health – can lead to a number of issues. Candida overgrowth can damage the gut wall and cause leaky gut (page 23).

Some common symptoms of candida overgrowth:

· Fatigue, especially after eating

· Diarrhoea and/or constipation

- Oral or vaginal thrush
- Fungal infections such as recurring tinea or athlete's foot, fungal nails, or an itchy scalp, nose or throat
- Gas and bloating, particularly after eating dairy, carbohydrates or fibrous foods
- Hypoglycaemia
- Mood swings, irritability and depression
- Adverse reactions to alcohol including red face, hangovers, personality changes or becoming intoxicated quickly after a small amount of alcohol
- Respiratory symptoms like hay fever or congested sinuses
- Skin conditions including acne, eczema, rashes, rosacea, psoriasis and hives
- Foul-smelling flatulence or sticky stools
- Sugar cravings, particularly after eating
- Worsening food sensitivities and intolerances

CONSTIPATION

Constipation can be an uncomfortable symptom of a number of underlying digestive issues, including leaky gut (page 23), general dysbiosis, food intolerances and some parasitic infections. But constipation can also be a stand-alone problem linked to dietary and lifestyle habits such as dehydration, a lack of fibre or exercise, chronic stress, the prolonged use of painkillers and some supplements (such as iron).

When we are constipated, the large intestine becomes filled with faecal matter that, over time, can cause pressure and injure the gut wall. Toxins that should be excreted are reabsorbed through the delicate gut lining before being recirculated back to the liver and kidneys. If these key detoxification organs become overburdened, the skin – the body's other elimination organ – must pick up the slack.

The ideal bowel motion should be smooth, well-formed and pass easily, without straining. Ideally, you should have at least one bowel motion per day.

You can improve symptoms quickly by implementing these simple techniques:

- *Rehydrate the bowels.* Start the day with 1–3 glasses of warm, filtered water with a generous squeeze of fresh lemon juice. In some traditional systems of medicine, warm water is recommended as it is thought to put less stress on the digestive system.

- *Rehydrate the body.* It's important to drink at least 6–8 glasses of filtered water daily. Consume 'wet' meals (soups, casseroles, stews) and watery foods such as fruit and vegetables to up your intake.

- *Minimise diuretics.* This includes alcohol, coffee, caffeinated tea and soft drinks.

- *Don't hold on.* When you feel the urge to pass a bowel motion, don't ignore it.

- *Eat regularly and chew well.* Chewing well allows your body to form a routine for elimination, releases digestive enzymes and helps the stomach break down what you've eaten, ultimately resulting in an easier bowel motion.

- *Consume 25–30 grams of fibre daily.* There are two types of fibre: soluble (found in oats, beans, apples, citrus, barley, lentils and psyllium) and insoluble (found mainly in vegetables and whole grains, nuts and seeds, and the skin of fruits), and both are essential for preventing constipation. Some soluble fibre dissolves in water, creating a gel-like substance, while insoluble fibre helps to bulk out stools and move things along. The key is to increase your intake slowly and drink plenty of water to avoid bloating and further constipation.

- *Exercise regularly.* Staying active helps massage the digestive tract and keep things moving. Try stretching, swimming, walking and yoga.

- *Massage the large intestine.* Lying on your back with your knees bent and feet flat on the floor, apply a small amount of oil to the skin over the belly and gently massage it, using circular clockwise motions, from the right hip up to under the ribs, then across the navel and down to the left hip.

- *Avoid laxatives.* Prolonged use of laxatives makes the bowel 'lazy', relying on the medicine to pass a bowel motion instead of the body's natural processes.

AUTOIMMUNE DISORDERS

Autoimmune conditions tend to have non-specific and chronic symptoms, which can be complex and difficult to diagnose, but they all have one thing in common: an immune response that causes the body to attack its healthy tissue. In recent years, there has been a huge spike in these conditions, which include rheumatoid arthritis, Hashimoto's and Grave's diseases, coeliac disease, psoriasis, type I diabetes and multiple sclerosis (to name but a few). This rapid growth indicates that our genes aren't solely to blame – rather, our modern diet and lifestyle may be wreaking havoc.

Our gut health plays an integral role in the prevalence of autoimmune conditions. Our microbiota protect our delicate gut lining – the body's defence against pathogens, toxins and bacteria. When our microbiota are out of balance, our likelihood of leaky gut (page 23) increases, triggering inflammation and taxing our immune system, which means we're less prepared to fight off infection and regulate this autoimmune response.

The good news is that there is building research on how to treat and manage these conditions, and gut health lies at the heart of it. Removing trigger foods such as gluten or casein can help to reduce gut inflammation, as can feeding your gut nourishing prebiotic- and probiotic-rich foods.

BLOOD SUGAR ISSUES

There is a multitude of factors that can contribute to blood sugar issues: if you eat something that causes your blood-sugar levels to rapidly spike, it causes a quick surge in insulin and may lead to inflammation in the gut. But our gut bacteria also play a key role in regulating our blood sugar. If our gut bacteria are out of balance, it can be challenging to keep blood-sugar levels stable[18]. Do you ever feel irritable, tired, experience headaches or have difficulty concentrating if you haven't eaten for a few hours? If so, you've likely felt the effects of a blood-sugar imbalance. To combat this, it's important to maintain a healthy, balanced microbiome. I also add a source of clean protein to my meals or snack on some nuts and seeds, which not only helps keeps me satiated, but ensures my blood sugar levels remain steady too.

OBESITY

Unfortunately, obesity has become an epidemic – both in Australia and across the developed world. While there are undoubtedly many factors that contribute to weight issues, the dramatic shift in our diet in recent years to one that is highly refined and processed is certainly one of the main culprits. The composition of microorganisms in the gut can affect nutrient absorption and energy regulation, therefore potentially leading to weight gain. Pre-clinical studies have shown that beneficial short-chain fatty acids, created by our microbes from the fibre we feed them in our diets, help regulate fat metabolism and may reduce a predisposition to weight gain. This fascinating field of research has already revealed how certain probiotic strains of bacteria can help to reduce gut inflammation and positively influence our metabolism[19]. Studies show how polyphenols – plant compounds found in a variety of wholefoods, herbs and spices – can help positively reset the microbiome and our metabolism and reduce our propensity to gain weight[20]. Interestingly, research shows that being exposed to antibiotics in the first few months of life, and a birth via Caesarean section, may also make us more likely to be overweight as an adult, as these factors can alter the microbial composition of the gut. As different bacteria can affect our natural tendency towards weight gain, by affecting how much energy we extract from our food as well as our blood-sugar levels and even our cravings, changing our diet can alter our microbial composition, and therefore reduce our chances of obesity[21].

The link between our gut health and our mood and overall sense of wellbeing is a complex one, but more and more research is helping us better understand the relationship between our gut and our brain. The gut–brain axis is very influential when it comes to our physical and mental health, and evidence shows that dysbiosis or inflammation in the gut can be a contributing factor of some mental illness, including anxiety and depression[22].

We tend to connect serotonin with happiness, but it also plays a role in gut motility, sleep, bone and cardiovascular health – and 90 per cent of it is produced in the gut[23]. Eating foods rich in tryptophan – such as eggs, nuts, seeds, cheese, lean meat and lentils – can help with serotonin production, which helps boost your mood. But if your gut isn't healthy, you probably aren't absorbing this vital nutrient. Leaky gut (page 23) changes the way some people's immune system cells in the brain work – they light up and are activated, which can interrupt the production and function of some neurotransmitters and impact our mental health[24].

Another neurotransmitter, gamma-aminobutyric acid (GABA), which helps reduce anxiety and stress and improves sleep, is produced by beneficial bacteria such as certain strains of *Lactobacillus*[25]. Consuming probiotic-rich, lacto-fermented wholefoods may be beneficial in helping to ease symptoms of anxiety[26].

The bottom line? While mood disorders, anxiety and depression are complex, nourishing your gut microbiome and reducing inflammation may be a helpful part of the management protocol.

If you're keen to understand more about your microbiome, you can take tests to get an overall picture. While tests can be helpful, they are not foolproof, and there is debate among practitioners about their accuracy, so it's wise to chat with a trusted GP or functional medicine practitioner to determine which ones may be of benefit to you.

- *Comprehensive stool test*. Sometimes referred to as 'complete digestive stool analysis', this test aims to determine the microbial diversity of your internal gut garden. Essentially, this test takes an overall snapshot of your gut health and indicates whether or not harmful bacteria, yeasts or parasites are present.

- *SIBO breath test*. This hydrogen and methane breath test determines whether SIBO (page 28) is present. These gases are produced by bacteria in the small intestine, so the test is used to measure whether or not these bacteria are contributing to gut issues. In the lead-up to the test, you're usually given a substrate such as lactulose to consume. It's not absorbed, so it simply acts as food for the bacteria, and as they ferment the lactulose they release gases that can then be measured.

- *Food allergy and sensitivity testing*. These tests help determine whether your body is making good immunological decisions. While there are many different types of food allergy tests, some of the more common ones include skin-prick testing and blood tests. If you've been eating well for a while but are still showing symptoms of impaired gut health, a cross-reactive food reactivity test may prove helpful. For example, people who are sensitive to gluten may experience similar symptoms after ingesting certain types of protein. This cross-reaction can trigger the immune system in the same way gluten does, so it's worth investigating if you're experiencing ongoing issues.

Understanding The Gut

HEALING THE BRAIN WITH GAPS

With growing evidence linking gut health issues to learning and behavioural issues like autism and ADHD, the GAPS (Gut and Psychology Syndrome) protocol, coined by Dr Natasha Campbell-McBride, aims to improve a patient's gut health in order to better the health of their brain[27]. Studies show that many patients with learning and behavioural difficulties have impaired gut health and nutrient deficiencies due to malabsorption. Dr Campbell-McBride suggests that people with autism, schizophrenia, and even depression and rheumatoid arthritis have difficulty digesting gluten and casein. This incomplete breakdown of the gluten protein results in the presence of gliadin peptides, which may have opioid effects and therefore act as an opiate on the brain.

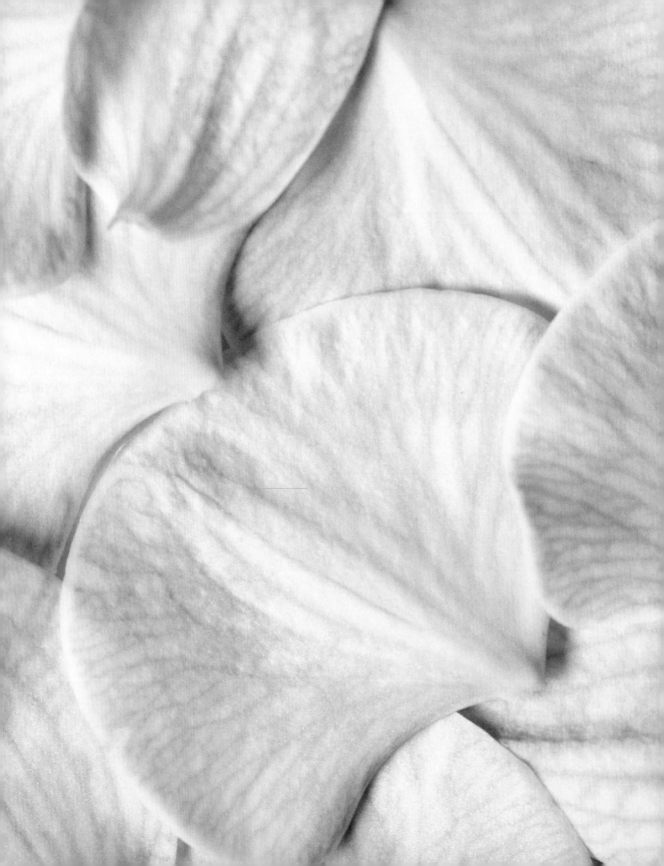

Is Your Skin Condition Caused By Your Gut?

The skin is a great barometer of what is going on inside the body. If your skin is irritated, inflamed or congested, chances are high that there may be an imbalance in your gut.

Our skin is our body's largest organ; it is one of the major systems by which the body expels toxins and waste and is our first line of defence against harmful bacteria and pathogens. Almost all skin conditions are linked to gut health, but diagnosing whether or not your skin condition is *caused* by digestive issues can be tricky. Sometimes the connection is obvious – for example, if drinking milk triggers indigestion, hives, a rash or eczema. Other times, the connection between our gut and our skin complaint can be more difficult to spot.

HOW DOES GUT HEALTH AFFECT THE SKIN?

In the same way our gut is in constant conversation with our brain (page 14), our gut has an intimate dialogue with our skin via the gut–skin axis[28]. This pathway allows the gut and skin to interact with one another, mainly via the microbiome. Many skin conditions have similar symptoms to gut conditions and the two are often closely linked and influenced by one another. So if our gut is out of balance, irritated or inflamed, our skin is one of the first places to exhibit symptoms. Research shows that up to 34 per cent of people suffering from irritable bowel syndrome (IBS) exhibit skin manifestations[29]. Leaky gut or intestinal permeability (page 23) can mean that our body is unable to absorb and use key nutrients, vitamins and minerals that are essential for strong, healthy skin. At the same time, if our gut is 'leaky' and LPS (endotoxins) are able to escape into our bloodstream, they are sent to the liver for processing. This places extra burden on the liver,

which is already dealing with our normal metabolic wastes and environmental and dietary chemicals. When the liver is overburdened, our skin takes on the responsibility of having to eliminate some of these toxins. Research shows that our gut health, as well as stress, can negatively impact the skin's protective antimicrobial barrier and make skin conditions worse[30].

To heal the skin, it's essential that you first heal the gut, fertilising it as you would a garden with essential nutrients and beneficial bacteria. More and more research supports the use of probiotics in the treatment of skin conditions, and these include species and strains from the genera of *Bifidobacterium*, *Lactobacillus* and *Streptoccocus*. Following are some common skin conditions that may be linked to the state of your microbiome and gut health.

ACNE

Unfortunately, acne and pimples don't discriminate, and, for many, they can be a source of embarrassment. Acne is a complex condition, so it's important to understand the underlying causes – they can either be hormonal or digestive, or a combination of both.

Hormonal acne: Raised hormone levels, or sensitivity to testosterone or other androgens, commonly contributes to acne. Too much testosterone in the body (or a sensitivity to it) stimulates sebaceous glands in the skin, causing oil production and clogged pores. Although this often occurs during puberty, it can also affect women mid-cycle or around their period when hormonal concentrations shift rapidly and oestrogen levels drop. Another acne-triggering hormone is cortisol, our stress hormone, which can affect the balance of bacteria in our gut, suppress our immune system and cause skin inflammation – enter acne.

Digestive acne: The close link between gut health, hormones and acne is an interesting one. Oestrogen and progesterone, for example, can affect the speed at which food is digested and moved along the digestive tract. This is why women, at various stages of their cycle, can experience bloating, diarrhoea and/or constipation. The gut also plays a key role in how oestrogen is eliminated by the body. When the elimination pathways are slowed down because of constipation, or the liver is overburdened due to a high level of toxins in the blood stream, oestrogen metabolism and elimination can be compromised and this can easily lead to hormonal imbalances.

Oestrogen dominance is a common condition that many women experience and the symptoms can worsen in the second half of their menstrual cycle. It essentially means that their oestrogen levels are too high in comparison to their progesterone. This can cause acne, along with premenstrual bloating, cramping, mood swings, sluggish metabolism, headaches, tender breasts and sugar cravings.

Other gut disorders, such as leaky gut (page 23) and SIBO (page 28), also have close links to acne. SIBO is ten times as prevalent in people with acne, and stress-induced leaky gut may contribute to local skin inflammation, which is seen in people with acne[31]. This cycle can be self-perpetuating, as an imbalance of bacteria or leaky gut can cause inflammation and malabsorption issues – meaning the skin isn't getting all the essential nutrients it needs.

ROSACEA

Rosacea is a chronic inflammatory skin condition characterised by redness or flushing, particularly over the cheeks and nose. Like with most skin conditions, there can be several triggers for rosacea: diet (hot and spicy foods, alcohol and caffeine) as well as hot temperatures or sun exposure, allergies, exercise and stress. Studies suggest that rosacea is also closely linked to gastrointestinal disorders and our intestinal bacteria. One study showed that patients with rosacea symptoms are also 13 times as likely to have SIBO (page 28)[32].

ECZEMA/ATOPIC DERMATITIS

Those who have suffered from eczema will understand just how complex, painful and debilitating it can be. This chronic skin condition can manifest as itchy, dry, patchy, or red skin and can cause immense distress. While there are thought to be countless triggers, the underlying cause of eczema is often leaky gut (page 23) or food allergies and intolerances.

Treatment, however, is not as easy as simply eliminating trigger foods. It is important to support immune function and a healthy inflammatory pathway. Gut health and microbial diversity also play a major role in the manifestation of eczema, also known as atopic dermatitis, as leaky gut and reduced microbial diversity can result in a weakened immune system – and a greater risk of skin inflammation and damage to the skin's protective barrier[33, 34].

This chronic autoimmune condition can cause dry, cracked, scaly and patchy skin. Like eczema, psoriasis is thought to be linked to leaky gut (page 23), because when endotoxins and other compounds leak through the gut wall, the body stages an attack, triggering an inflammatory response.

KERATOSIS PILARIS

Keratosis pilaris (KP) is a common skin condition – often referred to as 'chicken skin' – that appears as white or red bumps on the backs of the arms, thighs, buttocks, and sometimes the face. It is the result of a buildup of keratin (the protein that protects the skin), which blocks the hair follicle, resulting in lumps and bumps. While there's no definitive cause – and genetics may play a role – gut health is also a key factor, as many experts believe that keratosis pilaris is a result of nutrient deficiencies and malabsorption issues. Vitamin A is an important nutrient for a smooth, glowing complexion as it plays a major role in the healthy keratinisation of skin cells[35]. Those with KP are often deficient in it. Likewise, if you are struggling with malabsorption issues and have an essential fatty acid deficiency, you may be more prone to keratosis pilaris, as fatty acids are essential for combating skin inflammation. There is also a link between KP and gluten intolerance.

Our gut microbes do not age the way we do, per se. Our microbiome changes based on our lifestyle choices, diet and medications. As we get older, our gut microbes' capacity to produce anti-inflammatory short-chain fatty acids declines. This is because of our reduced capacity to support them due to changes in our bodies as we age, including an irregular transit time, reduced appetite and nutritional status.

Changes in the microbiome can result in dysbiosis, which has been linked to a range of age-related conditions and low-grade chronic inflammation. Low-grade chronic inflammation signifies one of the most consistent biologic features of ageing – and one of the main drivers for premature ageing of the skin and body. Our gut microbiota may be associated with inflammageing (ageing caused by inflammation), triggered by gut dysbiosis and weakened intestinal barrier function.

Pre-clinical studies have shown age-related deterioration of the gut barrier can occur, along with increased intestinal permeability and changes to the way the muscles of the digestive tract function. While we can't prevent the process of ageing, by promoting a healthy gut and gut microbiome, we may be able to slow down and reduce its negative effects.

Understanding The Gut

WHAT ABOUT POLYCYSTIC OVARIAN SYNDROME AND ACNE?

Polycystic ovarian syndrome (PCOS) is a condition that causes women to have higher than normal ratios of androgens (male hormones). Genetics can be a contributing cause, and insulin resistance and inflammation can be symptoms, as well as irregular menstrual cycles, male-pattern hair growth, weight gain, fertility issues, headaches and acne. If you suspect you have PCOS, chat with your GP about undergoing more rigorous hormonal tests.

How What We Eat Impacts Our Gut Health

Gut issues are both common and complex, but their increasing prevalence – as well as the skin and health conditions related to them – gives us cause to ponder how nutrition can play a key role in healing, and harming, the gut. It's essential to tend to your gut like you would a garden, feeding it nutrient-dense wholefoods. Here, we delve into some of the foods and components that can impact our gut, for better and for worse.

Allergies and sensitivities can be difficult to diagnose, as symptoms can be non-specific, but here are some to look out for:

Skin

- · Itchy, dry or flaky skin
- · Swelling or redness
- · Rashes
- · Pimples, pustules or whiteheads

Gut

- · Reflux
- · Bloating or flatulence
- · Anal irritation
- · Constipation and/or diarrhoea

Respiratory

- · Mucous
- · Wheezing
- · Chronic sinus congestion
- · Itchy eyes, nose and throat

Brain

- · Mental fogginess
- · Poor concentration
- · Dizziness

GLUTEN

In the evolutionary scheme of things, gluten is a relatively new protein in the human diet. As a result, our bodies don't have all the enzymes needed to properly break it down. Gliadin (a protein found in some grains, such as wheat) can be particularly damaging to the gut lining, aggravating the immune system as well as the skin. And you don't have to be coeliac to suffer the consequences. Non-coeliac gluten sensitivity (NCGS) is a condition that is neither autoimmune nor allergic in nature, yet produces symptoms similar to those seen in coeliac disease. According to preliminary research, consumption of gluten can stimulate the release of zonulin – a protein that triggers the tight junctions in the intestinal wall to open up, promoting leaky gut (page 23) and potentially leading to autoimmune disease in those who are genetically predisposed to it[36]. It's for this reason that a gluten-free diet is helpful for people already suffering from digestive issues, as well as for those looking to heal their gut.

DAIRY

There are two components in dairy that are known to cause gastrointestinal symptoms – lactose (the sugar component) and casein and whey (the protein component). Intolerances to dairy are usually attributed to lactose, but casein can also cause digestive upset. Fermented dairy products are easier to digest, as the bacteria have broken down some of the lactose.

FODMAPs are a collection of short-chain carbohydrate molecules – fermentable oligosac-charides, disaccharides, monosaccharides and polyols – found in many foods that prove difficult for some people to digest. When these molecules aren't thoroughly absorbed, they make their way down to the lower bowel. There they ferment, triggering gastrointestinal symptoms that are often attributed to irritable bowel syndrome (IBS): bloating, gas, abdominal pain, constipation, cramping and diarrhoea. Ongoing poor gut health can contribute to FODMAP sensitivities. The condition is tricky to diagnose because, for many people dealing with FODMAP sensitivity, they usually only react to one or two of them.

FODMAPs and the foods they are found in include:

- Fructans and oligosaccharides, found in wheat, onions, garlic and some legumes
- Disaccharides such as lactose, found in dairy
- Monosaccharides such as fructose, found in fruits, some vegetables and honey
- Polyols such as sorbitol and mannitol are naturally found in many fruits and vegetables and are sometimes used as sugar substitutes

The triggers and symptoms of IBS and FODMAP sensitivity vary, so it's best to chat with a qualified healthcare professional before embarking on a low-FODMAP diet – it can be very restrictive and involves eliminating a large number of foods before slowly reintroducing them. In saying that, the studies on the effects of such a diet are promising: up to 70 per cent of IBS sufferers maintained long-term symptom relief[37].

Fermentation and fermented foods are close to my heart – they're at the core of everything we do at The Beauty Chef and, in my opinion, are one of the simplest and most effective ways to support gut health and wellbeing.

Despite its recent surge in popularity, fermentation certainly isn't new. It has been around for thousands of years, used as a means of preserving food and adding flavour. Almost all traditional cultures have a history of fermentation, from kimchi in Korea to natto in Japan. Sauerkraut, cultured milk, miso, tempeh, kefir and kvass: they're all rich in beneficial bacteria and are delicious examples of fermented foods you can incorporate into your dishes at home. But the health benefits of the fermentation process extend far beyond a food's basic nutritional components.

Fermentation is a process where bacteria and/or yeasts are used to break down sugars and starches in foods. While there are many different methods of fermentation, over the years I've discovered lacto-fermented foods to be particularly beneficial for gut health and skin health. This method of fermentation predominantly uses the *Lactobacillus* species of bacteria and is shown to help the gut in a number of ways. It can improve the bioavailability of nutrients as well as provide the gut with a good dose of probiotic bacteria.

But the postbiotics produced as by-products of fermentation may be just as powerful when it comes to gut health. When probiotics feed on nutrients during the fermentation process, the 'waste' they leave behind are considered postbiotics, which research shows may help fight inflammation, maintain the integrity of the gut wall

Understanding The Gut

VEGAN & VEGETARIAN DIETS

There has undoubtedly been a movement of late towards plant-based diets, and there's no question that including more vegetables in our diet can improve our health. While a diverse diet full of fibre-rich fruits and vegetables can boost our microbiome and increase microbial diversity, a totally plant-based diet may place a different kind of stress on the gut by limiting the variety of foods and nutrients available to our bacteria. The recipes in our Gut Guide are versatile, many with options for those who want to eat vegetarian or vegan. Just remember that dietary diversity and balance are key.

and combat pathogens, as well as help modulate our immune system[38]. Aside from aiding digestion, fermented foods may alleviate symptoms of some inflammatory disorders and restore immune function.

While you can take over-the-counter probiotic supplements, they tend to only contain a few species or strains. Fermented foods are a naturally rich source of prebiotic foods, probiotics and postbiotics, which work together to support our health. If we think of food as medicine, then fermented foods are one of the most significant.

The potential benefits of fermented foods:

· They support intestinal mucosal barrier function, reducing the potential for toxins crossing the gut barrier and being absorbed into the bloodstream.

· Probiotics and postbiotics in fermented foods help balance and modulate the immune system by stimulating the secretion of certain immunoglobulins, T-cells and killer cells, and enhance phagocytic activity of macrophages. These cells keep the immune system in check by regulating inflammation, detecting foreign threats and destroying pathogens.

· Probiotics in fermented foods can secrete molecules that reduce inflammation of the digestive tract and help produce vitamins such as biotin, K and B12 – all great for skin health and overall health.

· They may improve bowel function and promote regularity, improving our detoxification capacity.

· Fermentation of foods helps break down complex molecules of the foods to allow for easier digestion.

PREBIOTICS

Prebiotics (non-digestible plant fibres) are resistant to digestion in the stomach and intestines, but are metabolised by bacteria in the colon. They help promote the growth and activity of beneficial bacteria and encourage a decline in pathogenic bacteria. Some research suggests that foods rich in polyphenols – micronutrients such as flavonoids found in plants – may exhibit prebiotic-like activity in the gut by increasing the levels of beneficial bacteria

and reducing the bad. For example, polyphenol-rich cacao can encourage the growth of the beneficial genera *Lactobacillus* and *Bifidobacterium*[39].

PROBIOTICS & POSTBIOTICS

Resistant to digestion in the stomach and the small intestines, probiotics are live bacteria that we consume, through foods and supplements, to support gut, immune health and overall wellbeing. Studies focused on the prevention and treatment of gastrointestinal diseases (such as irritable bowel syndrome) and inflammatory skin conditions, including eczema and dermatitis, have shown encouraging results regarding the use of probiotics.

A multitude of probiotics have been proven to have health benefits, and there are many we're only just learning about. Some of these genera include *Lactobacillus*, *Bifidobacterium*, *Saccharomyces*, *Enterococcus*, *Streptococcus*, *Bacillus*, *Akkermansia* and their associated species and strains. There's no one-size-fits-all approach and no 'perfect' probiotic profile guaranteed to work for everyone. Dr Holmes says that 'taking a probiotic supplement with high numbers of only one strain is arguably the opposite of taking care of our microbiome – from your microbes' perspective, it is a forced immigration program that they didn't get a say in'. The best thing you can do is eat a balanced diet and probiotic-rich fermented foods (that contain many different species and strains).

'Postbiotics' is a relatively new term that refers to the bio-active compounds produced by probiotic cells that are able to deliver health benefits through their activity on our immune system. These compounds are retained even after their parent cells (probiotics) are no longer alive. While this vein of research is new and evolving, we can experience these benefits by consuming fermented foods, where probiotics and postbiotics work in synergy to nourish our gut.

Dietary fibre is found primarily in vegetables, fruits, legumes, nuts and seeds, and it's one of the most important ways in which we can impact our microbial composition and influence our health.

As soluble fibre passes through the small intestine, it remains relatively unchanged until it arrives in the large intestine or colon. That's where it begins to ferment with the help of bacteria that possess carbohydrate-binding molecules and an extensive set of enzymes that allow for the hydrolysis (breakdown and digestion) of a wide variety of fibres[40]. The by-product of this fermentation process is short-chain fatty acids, which are vital for our gut, immune, metabolic and brain health. That is why researchers believe that a Mediterranean diet (characterised by a high intake of fruits and vegetables, legumes, a moderately high intake of fish and a lower intake of meat, dairy and alcohol) has such positive health outcomes.

When bacteria ferments fibre it changes your colon's pH, making it more acidic. Many pathogens are pH-sensitive, so this change in pH encourages levels of beneficial bacteria to rise and wards off harmful bacteria[41].

Pre-clinical research also shows that when microbes are starved of fibre, they may feed on the protein found in the mucosal lining of the gut, triggering inflammation and gut-related diseases. So getting enough fibre undoubtedly has health benefits, and not consuming enough can have adverse effects. With this in mind, here is a snapshot of the different types of fibre, their health benefits, and how to include them in your diet.

Soluble fibre: Soluble fibre attracts water, forming a thick gel in your intestines that slows digestion and helps you feel fuller for longer. Certain types, like oats (beta glucan) and psyllium, can also help stabilise blood-glucose levels and lower LDL cholesterol.

Foods high in soluble fibre:

· Fruits and some vegetables

· Legumes and beans (soaking will make them easier to digest)

· Nuts and seeds (soaking will make them easier to digest)

· Psyllium husk

· Oats

Insoluble fibre: This type of fibre doesn't dissolve in water, but rather absorbs it, creating 'bulk' that helps soften stools and promote regular bowel movements. A recent study found that insoluble fibres such as cellulose, which don't ferment as well in the gut as many soluble fibre sources, can increase gut transit rate, preventing the fermentation of non-digestible foods and helping to keep us regular[42].

Foods that contain insoluble fibre:

· Whole grains

· Unpeeled fruit and vegetables

· Cruciferous vegetables

· Leafy greens

· Root vegetables

· Onions

· Nuts and seeds (soaking will make them easier to digest)

With insoluble fibre, it's important not to overdo it. Despite its benefits, overconsumption leads insoluble fibre to bind to minerals in the gut, inhibiting absorption, and without enough water intake, it can have a constipating effect.

Fibre types best for the production of short-chain fatty acids in the colon:

· Arabinoxylan (cereal grains like wheat bran)

· Inulin (artichokes, garlic, leeks, onions, wheat, rye and asparagus)

· Fructooligosaccharides (bananas, onions, garlic and asparagus)

· Pectin (apples, apricots, pears, citrus and carrots)

· Resistant starch (grains, barley, rice that has been cooked and cooled, beans, green bananas, legumes and potatoes that have been cooked and cooled)

While most starch is digested in the small intestine, resistant starch travels to the large intestine where it is fermented by friendly bacteria to produce short-chain fatty acids. These acids are very important for helping to lower the pH of the bowel, which facilitates the proliferation of beneficial bacteria and helps keep the lining of the bowel healthy[43]. Resistant starch also absorbs fluid in the digestive tract and increases stool bulk, promoting regularity.

If you have symptoms that suggest your gut is out of balance, resistant starch may make your symptoms worse, so we suggest keeping its consumption to a minimum during stages 1 and 2 of the Gut Guide.

In the later stages, once your gut is feeling balanced, including more resistant starch in your diet will help provide fuel for your beneficial bacteria and foster a healthy microbiome.

SHORT-CHAIN FATTY ACIDS (SCFAS)

SCFAs such as acetate, propionate and butyrate are produced when dietary fibre is fermented in the colon. Butyrate has a multitude of benefits on the gut, including improved intestinal barrier function, inflammatory status, cell growth and differentiation, intestinal motility, immune regulation and iron absorption. An increase in lactic acid-producing bacteria results in a competition between beneficial and pathogenic bacteria for space and nutrients. Increased numbers of beneficial bacteria improve the mucosal integrity of the gut, aid nutrient absorption and production, and support immune, brain and metabolic health. Clinical studies show that not having enough butyrate-producing bacteria in the gut can lead to serious problems: ulcerative colitis, Crohn's disease, and even colorectal cancer. Fibre-rich fruits, vegetables and legumes help to encourage the production of SCFAs. For example, inulin (found in artichokes, leeks and asparagus) and pectin (found in apples, pears and citrus fruit) are great examples of the types of fibre that promote SCFA production.

How To Support The Gut

The gut is complex but also very resilient. With just a few weeks of nurturing and nourishing it, you can experience profound results. The question is: how do we heal, support and feed our gut?

There's no question that food is medicine, and that diet is the easiest way to influence our gut health.

Our Gut Guide program provides a comprehensive outline of how to heal, weed, seed and feed the garden that is your gut, and there are a number of ways you can support your gut health daily, both with your diet and beyond it.

WHAT WE EAT

Eat gut-healing foods. If you're looking to heal your gut, it's essential to consume nourishing foods that are gentle and soothing.

Choose foods that aid digestion. Certain foods can stimulate digestion and contain critical digestive-boosting enzymes: bitter greens such as dandelion, rocket (arugula), endive, chicory, and sour foods such as lemon, grapefruit and unpasteurised apple-cider vinegar. Fermented foods such as kimchi, sauerkraut, kefir and miso are also a delicious way to add flavour and aid digestion.

Avoid foods you are allergic or intolerant to. This may seem obvious, but it deserves emphasising: in order to heal the gut, it's essential to avoid any foods that you know you're allergic or sensitive to. This includes foods that cause your skin to flare up, as well as gluten, which is a common gut irritant (page 36 & 59). After completing the Gut Guide, you can slowly reintroduce these foods and monitor your reaction.

Eat home-cooked, nourishing meals. While eating at home isn't always possible, try to minimise how much you eat out, where you have far less control over the salt, sugar, additives and types of fat used in the cooking process.

Choose organic, seasonal and local produce, which is fresher and richer in nutrients. Organic produce is also free from nasties such as herbicides and pesticides, which may compromise gut health. Ensure you wash all produce before consuming it, especially anything that will be eaten raw.

Steam or sauté your vegetables. Raw vegetables and salads can be difficult for the gut to digest, and lightly steaming or sautéing them can help. We limit raw veggies until the later stages of the Gut Guide.

Eat a small amount of animal protein. There's no need to avoid animal protein when healing the gut, but be mindful of your portion sizes and frequency of consumption. To improve its digestibility, slice meat finely and marinate it in herbs and spices or a dressing containing papaya, pineapple or kiwifruit (which contain protein-digesting enzymes). Slow-cooked or braised meats are easier to digest, so drag out your slow cooker.

Don't be afraid to fast. We have naturally evolved to experience periods where food is scarce – fasting. While scientists are still trying to work out the optimal fasting period and how often we should do it, there is evidence to suggest that periodic fasting offers metabolic and microbiome benefits. When you don't eat for at least eight hours, fibre stays in your body long enough to give hardworking fibre degraders like *Bifidobacterium* time to enjoy it – and turn it into anti-inflammatory short-chain fatty acids such as butyrate (for more on fasting, see page 51).

HOW WE EAT

Although healing the gut begins with what we eat, it is also highly influenced by how we eat. There are several approaches to preparation and consumption that can improve digestion and assist in the gut-healing process.

Eat in a relaxed state. Make the time to sit down at the dinner table. Avoid eating on the run or while distracted by other activities, as you'll be more likely to rush and eat too fast. Take five to ten deep breaths before beginning your meal: this activates the parasympathetic nervous system, promoting a 'rest and reset' response rather than the adrenalin-dominant 'fight or flight' state, which can inhibit proper digestion.

Chew properly. If you chew your food slowly and carefully, putting your knife and fork down between each bite, you ensure your food is semi-liquefied before you swallow it. Digestion begins in the mouth, so chewing properly reduces the amount of work your digestive enzymes have to do once food reaches the stomach.

Maintain a consistent eating schedule. It's important to give your gut enough time between meals and snacks to digest food properly and reset. It takes food two to four hours to leave the stomach and five to six hours to completely leave the small intestine; if we eat before our previous meal has had a chance to leave the stomach, your body will always be digesting, forcing it to work constantly to produce digestive enzymes and other biological signaling agents. Pay attention to your hunger cues and aim for two to three meals a day, depending on whether or not you are fasting.

Avoid drinking large amounts of liquid with meals. This can dilute your gastric acids, making it more difficult for your body to digest foods and assimilate nutrients. If you absolutely must drink with your meal, take small sips of still warm or room-temperature water.

Minimise distractions. Avoid mindless eating by turning off the television and putting your smartphone away. Instead of worrying about work emails, take the time to enjoy your meal and engage with your friends and loved ones.

STRESS

When you consider the gut–brain connection, it's no wonder that chronic stress can negatively impact the balance and diversity of our gut microbiome. Interestingly, this connection works both ways: not only does stress impact our microbiota, but our microbiota can also affect our state of mind. While stress causes an unhappy gut, an unhappy gut also causes stress. The key is in learning to manage it.

Stress can affect the release of digestive juices and diverts blood away from the digestive tract into the muscles for fight or flight. Consequently, digestion takes longer and is less effective.

MEDITATION AND MINDFULNESS

Meditation is a great way to relieve stress and unwind, which is crucial for maintaining a healthy gut. Science is telling us that the impact of meditation on our health extends even further, actually influencing how our genes express themselves, particularly in relation to our body's inflammatory response[44].

Here are three ways to incorporate meditation and mindfulness into your daily life:

· Before setting off on your day, allow five to ten minutes to simply sit quietly and focus on your breathing.

- Practise mindful eating by taking a few minutes to breathe deeply before the beginning of each meal. Shift your awareness to your environment, taking in the sights and smells around you.

- Try a guided meditation class. It can be a great way to introduce the practice into your life, especially if you're unsure how to embark on meditation at home. There are many wonderful apps and online resources that can help you.

SLEEP

Gut health and sleep quality go hand in hand. Recent pre-clinical studies have shown that interruptions to the sleep cycle may disrupt the body's ability to maintain a healthy gut microbiome[45]. Conversely, the beneficial bacteria in your gut can boost your body's supply of melatonin, the hormone responsible for maintaining your sleep cycles. Melatonin also has a protective effect on stress-induced lesions in the gut, so maintaining a healthy sleep pattern is essential.

Important facts about sleep:

- Vitamin D plays an important role in sleep quality, so spend at least ten minutes a day in the sun, nature's best source! To avoid the UV peak of the day, early morning or late afternoon sun is best.

- Maintain a consistent sleep schedule, which will encourage your body to maintain a healthy flux of hormones according to when you need to go to sleep and when you wake.

- Avoid drinking caffeine late in the day. Instead, opt for herbal teas that induce relaxation such as chamomile, lavender and peppermint.

- Steer clear of screens and blue light before bed, which can affect your melatonin levels, or use a blue light filter for your devices.

- Exercise earlier in the day, as working out too close to bedtime can leave you wired rather than tired.

PERSONAL CARE

Although our gut health undoubtedly influences our skin – beauty begins in the belly, after all – our skin also has its own unique microbiome that helps protect us against infection and inflammation. Our skin is essentially our immune system's first line of defence. Unfortunately, many commercial skincare products, antibacterial soaps and abrasive cleansers can be problematic as they strip our skin of both pathogenic and beneficial bacteria. Our skin is porous, so any chemical we apply can potentially be absorbed into our bloodstream. While there are countless chemicals to look out for, some of the common offenders to steer clear of include parabens, synthetic colours or fragrances, phthalates and sodium lauryl sulfate (SLS). Opt for organic skincare products derived from botanical ingredients and wholefoods. A good rule of thumb: choose Certified Organic and if you can't pronounce it or wouldn't put it on your plate, don't put it on your skin!

TOXINS IN THE HOME

Maintaining cleanliness at home is important, but being *too* clean can actually have an adverse effect on our immune systems. Research indicates that exposure to a variety of microbes can train our immune systems how to react to bacteria in the environment and is key for the development and modulation of our immune system[46]. Harsh antibacterial cleaners designed to kill bacteria target beneficial as well as pathogenic bacteria, so steer clear of toxic chemicals and instead opt for natural, organic cleaning products. Better yet? Make your own cleaning products at home with baking soda, water, white vinegar and essential oils.

EXERCISE

According to recent studies, the health and diversity of our gut microbiome can be influenced by exercise.[47] In fact, exercise can increase the production of protective short-chain fatty acids. Aim for 30 to 45 minutes of low- to medium-intensity exercise daily: walking, yoga, pilates or bike riding. Just remember that more doesn't always equal better. High-intensity exercise can be beneficial to your health; however, we don't recommend it in Stages 1 and 2 of the Gut Guide while the gut is healing.

WATER

Other than keeping us hydrated, water essentially acts as a transportation system within the body, circulating beneficial nutrients and flushing out toxins and waste products. It is also especially important when it comes to consumption of soluble fibre, which is something we have included a lot in the Gut Guide diet. The trouble is that our tap water is treated, containing chemicals such as chlorine and fluoride, which, over time, may have an impact on our inner ecosystem. Aim for 2 to 3 litres (8 to 13 cups) of clean filtered water daily (based on body weight and physical activity). Always carry a bottle of water with you and eat naturally hydrating foods such as cucumber, lettuce, celery and green capsicum (bell peppers).

GARDENING MAKES YOU A BETTER HOST

Gardening isn't just a great way to get a little exercise in – it also exposes you to beneficial soil-based microbes that help build a more robust immune system and healthier microbiota. As so many of us live in urban environments, we're not exposed to as many soil-based organisms as our rural-dwelling friends. For a healthy gut, it's important to get outside as much as possible. Gardening is also a great way to grow your own organic fruits, vegetables and herbs free from harmful herbicides and pesticides.

In an interesting study that followed members of the Hadza tribe in Tanzania, researchers discovered that their microbiome and the balance of their gut bacteria actually shift seasonally due to changes in their diet and the seasonal availability of food[48]. According to the study, their guts are home to a unique microbial community, quite unlike that of any other modern human population. In fact, their traditional diet of plant roots, game and berries shows us what our ancestors' microbiomes might have looked like before the advent of agriculture and farming. But aside from the types of foods the Hadza eat, their environment and the way they eat play an important role too.

In other words, growing your own veggies and eating foods endemic to your area is a great idea – not only for the environment, but for your gut health.

PRACTISE GRATITUDE

Keeping a gratitude journal sounds time-consuming, but it is scientifically proven to improve your health. It's been shown to lower pain levels, stress hormones and blood pressure, boost motivation and optimism and improve your sleep and mood. A happy host makes for a happy microbiome. Start by writing down three things you are grateful for each night. Show your gratitude to others by sending them a card or giving them a call to say thank you. Or simply spend time outdoors and appreciate the beauty of nature.

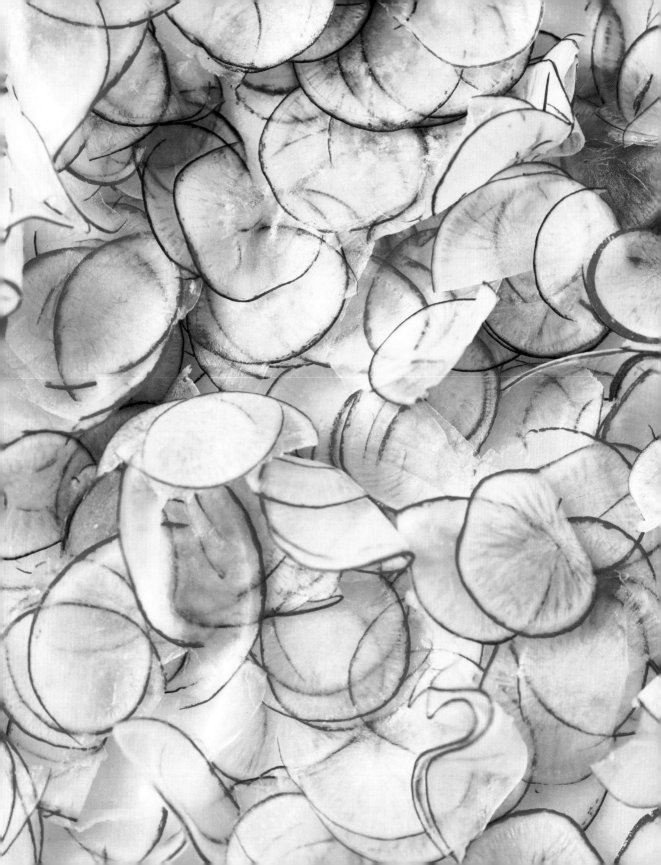

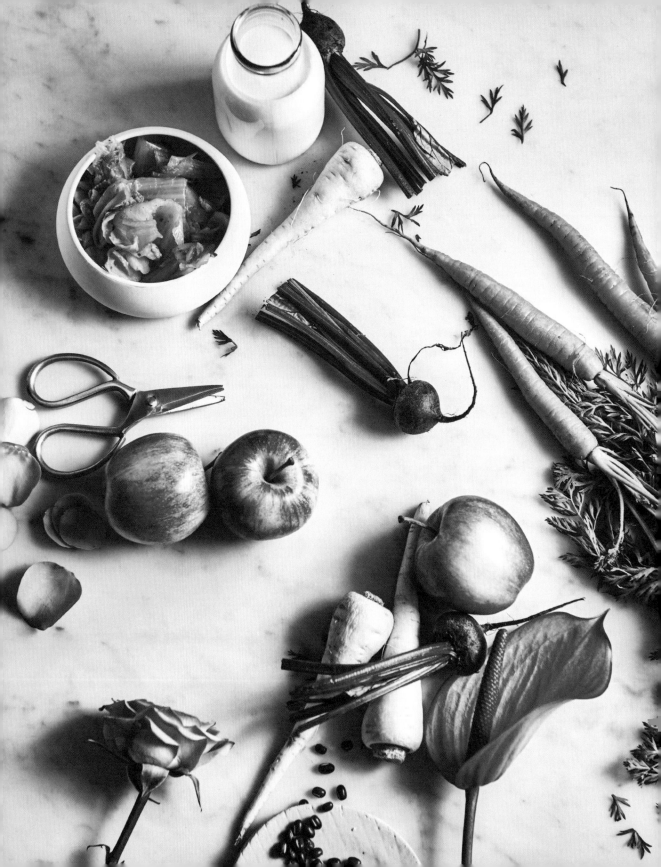

Part 2

The Beauty Chef Gut Guide

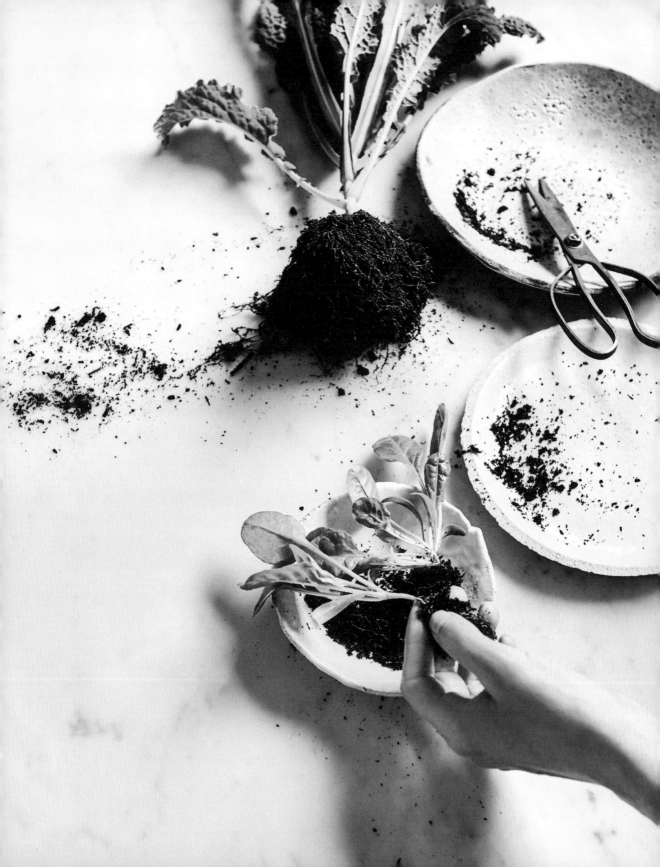

Look After Your Gut, Be Gutsy
& Follow Your Gut Instinct

The Beauty Chef Gut Guide program has been designed to provide you with the knowledge, tools and delicious recipes you need over eight weeks to help heal, weed, seed and feed your gut and nurture your microbiome. Whether you suffer from a specific gut issue, your complexion isn't as radiant as you would like it to be, or you simply feel that your digestion is unbalanced and you are lacking energy and vitality, this holistic, comprehensive guide will take you through four vital stages to help restore your gut health and overall wellbeing. It's important to remember that this is a general guide – your microbiome is unique, so if something doesn't feel right, then listen to your gut. This may mean staying in a certain stage for longer, or not eating a food recommended in a stage if it causes discomfort or unease.

While all the recipes in the Gut Guide are made of healthy wholefoods that are beneficial for gut health, if your gut is out of balance, even some 'healthy' foods can cause discomfort and aggravate your condition. That is why we have created stages, so you can ease your way into good gut health.

If you are experiencing persistent health issues, consult with a qualified health care practitioner before starting the Gut Guide program to determine what the underlying causes are.

STAGE 1: HEAL (2–4 WEEKS)

This stage focuses on soothing and calming your digestive system and bringing your diet back to the basics. By removing gluten, dairy, high-FODMAP foods and common allergens, and introducing foods that help calm your gut (and are a little easier to tolerate), your digestive system is given the break it needs to heal.

2: WEED (2 WEEKS)

This stage follows on from the two to four weeks you'll have spent healing your gut in Stage 1. While remaining gluten and dairy free (and still a little basic), Stage 2 introduces foods that help 'weed out' the bacteria we don't want and stimulate digestive enzymes so you can digest your food more efficiently. It is still a good idea to stick with simple, non-irritating foods as weeding can be a little stimulating to your digestive system.

STAGE 3: SEED (2 WEEKS)

After a few weeks of bringing your digestive system back to a 'blank canvas', it is time to introduce pre- and probiotic foods to boost beneficial bacteria, promote microbial diversity and help maintain a healthy digestive environment. In this stage, we add fermented foods, more polyphenol-rich fare, prebiotic-rich vegetables and some seeds and nuts, while following the principles learnt in Stages 1 and 2. By slowly introducing foods that may once have triggered symptoms, you may be able to better tolerate them.

STAGE 4: FEED (2 WEEKS)

Now that the soil is healthy and you've planted the seeds (probiotics), it's time to water them. We add more prebiotics and some resistant starch, which act as a 'fertiliser' for the beneficial bacteria in your gut. Prebiotic dietary fibres pass through the small intestine undigested and go straight to the large intestine to feed the beneficial bacteria. We also add more raw foods as well as seeds and nuts.

Gut-Loving Protocol

You can boost your digestion throughout the program with these tips:

1 Have a shot of Bone Broth (page 229) each morning: it's full of amino acids that help repair your gut lining.

2 Before meals, chew on bitter leaves such as endive, chicory or radicchio, or ginger or parsley, which aid digestion by stimulating digestive enzymes. Alternatively, have a shot of lemon juice or unpasteurised apple-cider vinegar (2 teaspoons of either in half a glass of warm water) half an hour before meals.

3 Eat appealing food. The smell of delicious, appetising food stimulates digestive juices even before we eat. This priming process is less likely to happen with unappealing food.

4 Eat when you're hungry and stop when you're full. Hunger signals that our digestion is ready for food, while eating when not hungry can overtax the digestive process. It's equally important to avoid overeating, which can cause the gastric juices and enzymes that assist digestion to become depleted, leaving you feeling full and bloated. Think of the stomach like a wood fire: too much wood will smother the fire.

5 Don't eat late at night. During sleep, digestion virtually stops. If you don't feel like breakfast on waking, you're probably eating too late and the food isn't being digested properly. Try having a very light meal to see if you feel different in the morning. You'll notice that your sleep improves and you have fewer vivid dreams.

6 Eat a diverse, balanced diet, and everything in moderation. By giving your bugs a varied diet, your gut reaction will be minimised if something is irritating.

7 Aim to have more plants on your plate than meat – this proportion is far healthier for promoting microbial health.

8 Eat more omega-3 fats and consume saturated fats like ghee, butter and coconut oil, but in moderation. While these saturated fats have health benefits and are healthier to cook with than refined vegetable oils, too much may upset your microbiome. Enjoy cold-pressed olive oil liberally on salads.

9 Go slow and don't overexercise. Stress and exercise can be taxing on our digestive system, so take it easy and keep your exercise regular, but moderate.

10 Remember the gut-brain axis. Breathe clean air, get involved with nature, garden, walk, meditate, practise gratitude and have fun.

General Principles
Of The Gut Guide Program

The table on pages 53–57 provides a list of what foods to enjoy and avoid while using the Gut Guide, and in general when caring for your gut. Just remember to take into account the specific guidelines for each stage (pages 59–62, 66–7, 70 and 73).

All of the foods we suggest you enjoy have properties that help heal, calm and restore gut health. Each ingredient has been chosen for its anti-inflammatory and/or antioxidant activity as well as nutritional value. You'll find a diverse range of wholefoods high in fibre, protein, healthy fats, vitamins and minerals, aimed at healing the gut wall and increasing microbial diversity.

If you suffer from any allergies, intolerances to or known digestive issues with any of the foods listed in the 'Enjoy' column, please avoid them. If there are ingredients that you discover cause discomfort, simply cut them out until a later stage before trying them again.

As a general rule, follow these principles for the duration of the Gut Guide program:

- Avoid processed foods and stick to low-HI (human intervention) foods: look for organic, free-range, grass-fed, fresh and unprocessed.

- Avoid refined sugars and high-GI (glycaemic index) foods. Refined sugar causes dysbiosis and inflammation in the body. Limit natural sugars found in fruits, honey and pure organic maple syrup. Remember, you're sweet enough!

- Avoid unfermented dairy and gluten, corn and unfermented soy for the duration of the Gut Guide and consider limiting them beyond the Gut Guide program.

- Remember, we offer healthy snack ideas as an option, but recommend that you don't overeat as this puts stress on your digestive system. Its important to eat according to your body weight, exercise routine, health status and hunger levels.

FASTING

We encourage you to practise the art of resting, not only your body and mind but also your hard-working digestive system. Intermittent fasting, which is characterised by cyclic periods of fasting and non-fasting during a defined period, is a great way to do this. This method of eating has received increased attention for its ability to affect the human microbiome. Some pre-clinical animal studies suggest that time-restricted feeding can induce changes in the gut microbiome, contributing to the diversity of our microflora, and that fasting strengthens the gut barrier and activates the molecular pathway by which our brain communicates with the gastrointestinal tract[49].

By strengthening our gut lining and giving our digestion a little break, fasting may be an effective tool in restoring gut health. While there are varying opinions regarding optimal fasting regimes, such as length of fasting interval, number of fasting days per week and recommendations for dietary behaviour on fasting versus non-fasting days, it is important to be aware that everyone is different and should find a routine that works best for their condition. We suggest consulting with your healthcare professional before adopting fasting.

If you do wish to add a day or two of fasting while on the Gut Guide, Crescendo Fasting is considered the gentlest approach. It involves fasting on two to three non-consecutive days a week during a 12- to 16-hour window. For example, if your last meal was dinner at 6 pm, your first meal the following day would be between 6 am and 10 am. Fasting for 16 hours will give your digestive system more of a rest, but working your way up from 12 hours is a good way to ease into it gently. It is also recommended that exercise be kept to a minimum on fasting days (think yoga and leisurely walks) and, as always, drink plenty of water.

While we recommend spending two to four weeks in the Heal stage and 2 weeks each in the Weed, Seed and Feed stages, please be aware that this is a general guide and will vary depending on your condition. You may need to stay in each stage for a while longer, depending on your issues.

How do you know if it's time to move from Stage 1 to Stage 2? Ideally, your gut will feel calmer, less bloated and generally less symptomatic. If this isn't the case, then you should spend more time in Stage 1 before graduating to Stage 2. As a general rule, if the gut is soothed and calm before starting any kind of treatment for parasites or dysbiosis, the side effects will be minimised and treatment will be more effective.

Whether you are working with a practitioner to correct dysbiosis using herbs and nutrients, or are simply introducing naturally anti-parasitic and antifungal foods as per our guidelines, it is not unusual to experience stronger symptoms in Stage 2 as your body is essentially in a state of detox. If you feel that your gut is irritated, bloated, sore or you are having more frequent, urgent bowel movements, then we recommend you remain in Stage 2 before continuing to Stage 3. If you are under the guidance of a practitioner, they may slow the process down and let your gut adjust to the effects of the anti-parasitic treatment before continuing.

Below is a list of possible symptoms you may experience in Stage 2, or more generally throughout the course of the guide, and what to do about them.

Symptoms	What to do
Bloating and gas	It is normal to have some bloating and gas throughout the Gut Guide. If it becomes more intense, you may want to ease up on some of the more potentially 'active foods', such as fermented foods and cruciferous vegetables.
	Increase fluid intake and ensure you have at least one daily bowel motion. Warm fluids such as herbal teas and broth can be very effective in inducing them.
	If symptoms do not ease, you may need to repeat Stage 1 and work on calming the gut for longer before moving back to Stage 2. While a small amount of gas production is part of the normal digestive process, it shouldn't be excessively smelly, in great volume or cause you pain. Check with your health care practitioner if any symptoms persist.
Detox symptoms, which may include: Fatigue Headaches Skin breakouts Mood changes/irritability Body aches	You may experience these symptoms at any stage of the Gut Guide. The diet removes many difficult to digest, harmful or allergenic foods such as sugar, caffeine, gluten and dairy. This can cause some people to experience symptoms similar to that of a detox – this is completely normal, and just means that the process is working. If you experience discomfort, cut down on some of the more challenging/stimulating foods and reintroduce them in a week's time, but more slowly. These symptoms can be signs of other medical issues, so please always check with your health care practitioner.

Foods To Enjoy & Foods To Avoid

	Enjoy	Avoid as much as possible	Foods only allowed at certain stages of the Gut Guide
Vegetables	Most cooked vegetables can be eaten freely from Stage 2 (unless you are continuing on a low-FODMAP diet). Some are only allowed during specific stages (see the third column).	Corn (a common allergen and high glycaemic).	Potatoes are high in resistant starch when boiled and cooled. We include them in Stage 4. Opt for low-GI varieties such as Nicola and Carisma.
	Organic seaweed and sea vegetables	Mushrooms (they can carry mould).	Raw vegetables are enzyme-rich, nutrient-dense foods, but if the gut is very irritated then avoid until it has calmed and digestion has improved. Eat vegetables steamed or sautéed instead.
	Olives (in brine), in moderation	Pre-packaged vegetable juices	
	Tomato paste and tomato passata (puréed tomatoes) in glass jars	Tinned vegetables	
	NOTES		Raw vegetables in smoothies and freshly pressed juices may be tolerated, but sip slowly and swish liquid around the mouth before swallowing. For those who find raw vegetables difficult to digest, try lightly steaming before adding them.
	Buy organic fruit and vegetables whenever possible.		
	All vegetables need to be washed well in filtered water.		Fermented vegetables (using salt) or commercially fermented vegetables (using a starter culture) can cause gas and bloating if the gut is imbalanced. Introduce them slowly.
	Non-organic vegetables need to be scrubbed really well and peeled wherever possible.		
	Certain vegetables should always be eaten organic, including carrots, potato and broccoli, due to intensive and concentrated spraying.		Tinned tomatoes are okay for occasional use, but look for organic ones in BPA-free tins. Better still, use chunky tomato passata (puréed tomatoes) in glass jars in place of tinned tomatoes.
Fruit	Lemons	Fruit juice that is commercially prepared, reconstituted and stored on a shelf with preservatives.	Dried fruit. Ensure they are preservative free and ideally organic. Enjoy in moderation from stages 3 & 4 onwards.
	Limes		
	2 of the following are allowed daily: ½ cup fresh or frozen berries (raspberries, blackberries, blueberries; organic if frozen); 1 apple, pear, nectarine, peach, apricot, plum; ½ small papaya, ½ banana.	Fruit that is prone to mould (melon, grapes).	All fruit juices are high in carbohydrates and have a high glycaemic index. A green apple may be juiced with vegetables and enjoyed occasionally.
		Fruits that have a high glycaemic index (grapes, mango).	

	Enjoy	Avoid as much as possible	Foods only allowed at certain stages of the Gut Guide
Meat (in moderation)	Free-range and/or organic chicken and turkey Red meat (including game meat) can be eaten 1–2 times per week, if desired. Lean lamb is best. Lean beef is okay for some, but should be avoided if you have an inflammatory skin condition. Organic and grass-fed meat is preferred, but if not possible, aim for grass-fed.	Processed deli meats like ham, sausages, bacon, etc.	Meat cooked at high temperatures (barbecue, pan fried): eat in moderation. Organic minced/ground meat is okay, but some reports suggest that the commercially prepared variety can have higher levels of bacteria contamination, so it would be best to mince your own from organic meat, or ask your butcher to do it fresh for you.
Seafood	Fish, fresh only (see 'Avoid' list) Choose wild-caught, deep-sea, cold-water oily fish where possible; sardines are ideal. Fresh, wild-caught salmon: farmed salmon contains chemicals, preservatives and dyes. NOTE If you cannot source a particular wild-caught fish variety, substitute for an easy-to-source one.	Fish high in mercury: swordfish, king mackerel, tilefish or golden tile, flake, shark or orange roughy Prawns, oysters, mussels, lobster, crab, etc. Processed fish products (smoked salmon, fish fingers, etc.) Farmed salmon from farms that use antibiotics.	Salmon farmed without the use of antibiotics is okay if you can't find wild-caught salmon. Occasional tinned fish is okay (sardines, red salmon, tuna). Opt for BPA-free tins.
Grains	Gluten-free 'pseudo' grains: amaranth and buckwheat are allowed throughout the Gut Guide, but should be soaked to decrease phytic acid. Quinoa is also allowed but should be rinsed thoroughly before cooking.	Wheat and all wheat products Soy flour Rye, barley, spelt, kamut and any other gluten-containing grains.	White basmati rice is low GI and low FODMAP at 1 cup (190 g/6½ oz) of cooked rice. If you have an issue digesting cauliflower rice or are not a fan of quinoa, you can swap them out for basmati from Stage 2 onwards. Eat in moderation and keep serving sizes within the low-FODMAP range. I prefer to use white basmati rice, rather than brown, as it is easier to digest. To prepare, soak overnight in water and rinse thoroughly. Cook in 5 times the amount of water until tender. Drain and rinse with hot water. Gluten-free oats can be introduced from Stage 4.
Legumes	Tempeh is okay to consume during the Gut Guide as it is fermented. Chickpeas, kidney beans, lentils, cannellini beans, butter beans, adzuki beans, black beans (no more than ½ cup per day), soaked and cooked fresh, can be enjoyed from Stage 2. NOTE If the gut is very irritated, avoid legumes until it has calmed and digestion has improved. If you are low FODMAP, use tinned legumes.	Textured vegetable protein (TVP) Soy milk, soy yoghurt, soy cheese Soy flour Soy oil	Tofu is unfermented soy, therefore we recommend consuming it in moderation. If you are vegan and are limited with protein choices, then it can be eaten 1–2 times per week. GM-free and organic tofu is best.

	Enjoy	Avoid as much as possible	Foods only allowed at certain stages of the Gut Guide
Eggs	Fresh, organic free-range eggs (stored in the fridge) NOTE The ideal way to cook eggs is to avoid exposing the yolk to air, which prevents oxidation of the good yolk fats. This includes poaching under water and soft boiled.	Non-organic eggs	
Dairy & milk alternatives	Unsweetened almond milk, macadamia milk, drinking coconut milk and UHT coconut milk. Fresh coconut and nut milk are always best. NOTE Use unsweetened UHT coconut milk if you are on a low-FODMAP diet. Tinned coconut milk and cream, coconut yoghurt and coconut water. If possible, buy BPA-free tins and choose brands that don't add guar gum, sugar or any other additives to the coconut milk. Organic, grass-fed and cultured butter (lactose is converted to lactic acid in the culturing process, making it easier to digest). Organic, grass-fed ghee (see page 62)	Milk, cream, ice cream, sour cream and most cheeses.	Small amounts of sheep's and goat's cheese and yoghurt, if tolerated.
Fats & oils	Organic, grass-fed cultured butter Organic, grass-fed ghee for high-temperature cooking. Extra-virgin olive oil for cooking and drizzling over salads and vegetables. Extra-virgin coconut oil for low-temperature cooking. Macadamia and avocado oil for low-temperature cooking. Cold-pressed flaxseed oil: raw form only, and in small amounts as a daily supplement if desired.	Margarine Deep-fried foods Reheated oils Vegetable oils (sunflower, safflower, corn, soy) Peanut oil Refined sesame oil Any other oil not listed in the 'Enjoy' column.	Ghee or refined coconut oil for high-temperature cooking (use this cooking method only occasionally).
Spreads, sauces & toppings	Nut butters (not peanut) Tahini (hulled, unhulled and black)	Jam, peanut butter, cheese and other commercially made spreads. Commercially prepared salad dressings and mayonnaise. Commercially prepared sauces (tomato, barbecue, chilli, etc.). Mustard that is highly processed and contains preservatives and additives (American mustard and dijonnaise).	Small amounts of organic and preservative-free mustard can be used in homemade sauces and salad dressings. High-quality, organic artisan sauces and dressings are okay (carefully read labels).

	Enjoy	Avoid as much as possible	Foods only allowed at certain stages of the Gut Guide
Nuts & seeds	Nuts and seeds are best eaten after they have been soaked and dried. Soak them in warm water with sea salt, a ratio of 1 cup nuts/seeds to 1-2 teaspoons* of sea salt, soaking for at least 7 (and up to 12) hours. Drain and rinse, then dry out using a dehydrator or in the oven at 60°C (140°F) for 12-24 hours, or until dry. NOTES Adding sea salt to the soaking water releases enzymes (phytase) present in nuts and seeds that in turn reduce phytic acid, which can impair digestion. Drying them helps reduce any further phytic acid and makes them perfect for storing. Buy small amounts and use them quickly. Store all nuts and seeds in the fridge or freezer to prevent them from going rancid. *Pumpkin seeds (pepitas) and sunflower kernels require 2 teaspoons of salt.	Peanuts All roasted nuts Salted nuts Peanut butter Pistachios and cashews, as they are more prone to growing mould.	NOTES Although nuts and seeds are introduced from Stage 2 onwards, those following a vegan diet may feel they need to add them in Stage 1 as a protein-rich snack. All nuts and seeds must be raw and unsalted and should be limited to ten per serve unless otherwise stated. If your gut is very irritated, avoid whole nuts and seeds until it's calmed and digestion has improved. Instead, eat ground nuts or nut butters. Walnuts, almonds and macadamia nuts have the best fatty acid profiles. You can also have pecans, hazelnuts and Brazil nuts. Pumpkin seeds (pepitas), sunflower kernels, chia and hemp Linseed/flaxseed (freshly ground at home, stored in the fridge and eaten quickly)
Sweeteners		Artificial sweeteners Agave Table sugar Corn syrup Fruit sweeteners	Use the following in moderation: Stevia, Xylitol Raw organic honey Pure organic maple syrup Blackstrap molasses Coconut sugar Small quantity of organic dates, dried sulphur-free apricots and raisins.
Beverages	Filtered water Green tea (max 2 cups daily) Herbal teas Drinks from the Tonics & Healing Elixirs chapter (page 83)	Tap and/or bottled water Soft drinks and/or cordials Alcohol Coffee, black tea NOTE If you must have coffee, choose organic and black or with almond milk. No added sugar/flavourings. But ideally, try to go without.	Natural sparkling mineral water (occasionally, and not with meals).
Processed & convenience foods		Processed junk foods Unhealthy fast foods Convenience/frozen meals	Some foods can be bought ready-made, such as hummus, nut spreads and healthy dips. Make sure they do not contain preservatives, colourings, additives, flavours or sugars.

	Enjoy	Avoid as much as possible	Foods only allowed at certain stages of the Gut Guide
Seasoning, condiments & flavourings	Homemade bone or vegetable broth Apple-cider vinegar (raw, organic, unfiltered, fermented and unpasteurised) Fresh lemon and lime juice Organic tamari and shoyu Fresh herbs and spices Ground herbs and spices that are stored away from moisture and light (replace regularly to prevent mould). Celtic and Himalayan sea salt Freshly ground pepper Raw cacao powder Coconut aminos Natural (pure, organic) vanilla extract (for an alcohol-free alternative, use vanilla powder at half the recipe quantity as it is very concentrated). Nutritional yeast	Soy sauce (contains gluten) Distilled vinegars Preservatives Colourings and flavourings 200 numbers (sulphites) 600 numbers (MSG) Textured vegetable protein (TVP) Commercially prepared stocks, gravies and sauces	High-quality, organic pre-prepared stock and bone broth (carefully read the labels for additives, sugar, salt). Fresh, minced and dried garlic, ginger and chilli (be careful of added preservatives, sugar and salt if commercially minced). Organic miso paste
Cooking & soaking methods	Steamed Lightly boiled Marinated or slow-cooked animal proteins NOTE Pair animal proteins with tropical fruit such as pineapple or papaya (the enzymes will help break protein down, making it easier to digest).	Fried/deep-fried	Baked/roasted Grilled/barbecued at low temperatures; be careful not to blacken the food at all. Limit raw vegetables until later stages of the Gut Guide. Soak chickpeas in warm water with bicarbonate of soda (baking soda) for 12 (and up to 24) hours. Drain, rinse and change the water and bicarb 1-3 times during the soaking period. Soak puy, green and brown lentils in warm water with a splash of unpasteurised apple-cider vinegar or lemon juice for 7 hours (and up to overnight). Drain, rinse and change the water and acid medium 1-2 times during the soaking period. All other legumes require a longer soaking time of 12 (and up to 24) hours. Adding kombu to the cooking water of legumes and pulses helps break down the raffinose sugars (which release carbon dioxide and hydrogen, causing uncomfortable gas), making them easier to digest and their nutrients more available to absorb.

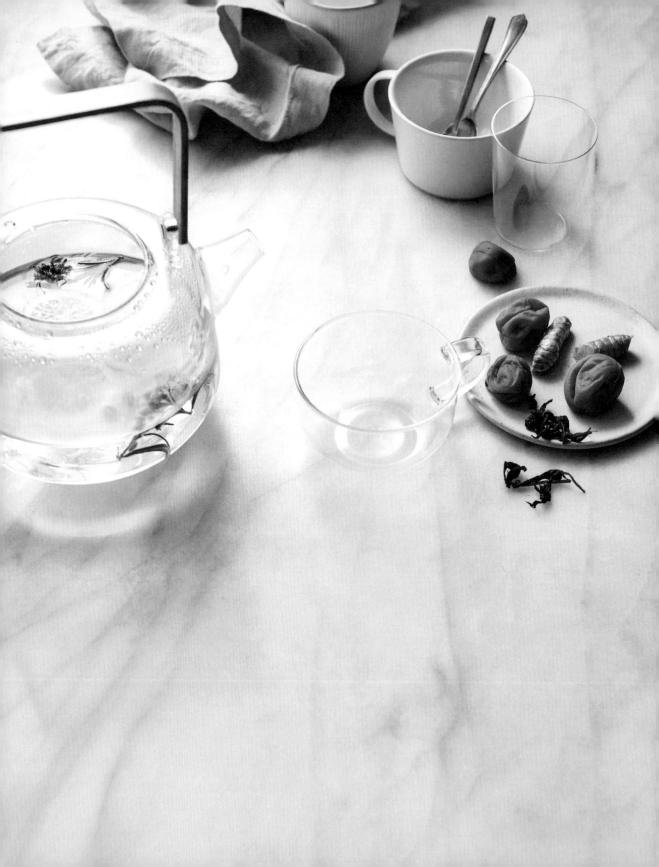

Stage 1: Heal

Week 1, 2 & Onwards If Needed

The first stage of the Gut Guide focuses on bringing your diet back to basics. In this stage, we remove all processed foods and potential irritants, including gluten, dairy, high-FODMAP foods and allergens. We focus on foods that help calm the digestive system and give it the break it needs to focus on healing.

While we recommend a minimum of two weeks in this stage, your gut may need longer to heal, especially if you suffer from SIBO, IBS or leaky gut syndrome. In this case, we recommend working alongside your health practitioner, who will help determine when you are ready to move to Stage 2. Your practitioner will also be able to help further tailor your diet to suit your condition, as there may be some foods that, while great for your gut, could trigger symptoms if your condition is advanced.

NEED A BOOST?

If you do not suffer from an advanced gut disorder and have no serious symptoms, but feel that your gut and body could do with a reboot and your skin could look more 'glowy', you can follow Stage 1 with less restriction, including recipes labelled with the 'Stage 2 Friendly' tag two to three times a week. These recipes are still gluten and dairy free, and easy on your digestion, but they include cruciferous vegetables, insoluble fibre and some FODMAPs. While we have not specifically included fermented vegetables in Stage 1, these can be included if well tolerated. We allow a small amount of probiotic coconut yoghurt in Stage 1 and coconut milk kefir in Stage 2. These types of fermented ingredients will be introduced in larger quantities in Stage 3.

It's important to remember that if you've turned to our Gut Guide, chances are your gut is inflamed, irritated and not functioning to its full potential, or you are experiencing skin issues (a good sign your gut is out of balance). It is essential to take the time to heal and calm your digestive system using the guidelines that follow.

IDENTIFYING TRIGGER POINTS

The first step in any elimination diet is to remove the two most common allergenic and gut-irritating foods: gluten and dairy. In many cases, this can calm a multitude of gut symptoms such as gas, bloating, discomfort, alternating bowel motions, etc. However, if you are still experiencing gut problems – and they appear to be random and don't follow any pattern – you may be sensitive to a natural food chemical. The most common ones are histamines, amines, salicylates, oxalates and glutamates. These are found in many healthy foods, and symptoms can be varied and debilitating. Symptoms may include neurological issues (headaches and irritability), low energy and fatigue, respiratory and skin issues (itchiness, hives, rashes) and more.

There are a number of underlying causes for such intolerances, and it's very difficult to avoid natural chemicals in the diet as they are abundant in many of the healthiest fruits and vegetables. It's never a good idea to attempt to remove them from your diet without the guidance of a health care practitioner. Another important step is to address the underlying cause – often a disrupted gut function and microbiome.

Low FODMAP: In a person with healthy gut function, many FODMAP foods are beneficial, acting as prebiotics that stimulate the growth of healthy gut microbes. However, if you are suffering from a digestive disorder or your gut is imbalanced, these same foods can induce symptoms such as gas, bloating, irregular bowel movements and pain. For this reason we will stick to low-FODMAP foods in Stage 1, reintroducing some beneficial FODMAP-containing ingredients in later stages. (However, if you are specifically intolerant and have been advised by a practitioner to remain on a low-FODMAP diet, we suggest following these guidelines for the remainder of the program.) There are many important FODMAP vegetables that should not be taken out of the diet for long periods of time, including cruciferous vegetables. They contain some very important anticancer nutrients and are crucial to a healthy diet. Remember that a low-FODMAP diet is not a long-term treatment for a gut condition. It should be used short-term to give symptom relief and calm the gut, but the underlying problem needs to be corrected.

Low allergen: Food allergens are naturally occurring compounds in foods that can cause an inflammatory immune response. Peanuts, tree nuts, milk, eggs, sesame seeds, shellfish, fish, soy and wheat contain common allergens. Although eggs are an allergen for some people, we will be keeping these in Stage 1 as they are a good source of protein and high in choline, which is great for fighting inflammation and generally cannot be synthesised in the body alone, so it is essential that we get it from the foods we eat. We will also be including fish in this stage as it is a good source of protein and high in anti-inflammatory compounds. If you have an allergy or intolerance to fish or eggs, continue to exclude these from your diet. Nuts, seeds and fermented dairy will be reintroduced in Stage 2, provided you don't have an allergy or intolerance.

Limit cruciferous vegetables (for now): This group of vegetables, which includes broccoli, cauliflower, brussels sprouts, kale and cabbage, is high in raffinose, an oligosaccharide that the human body cannot break down. Raffinose passes through the small intestine undigested and travels to the large intestine where it is anaerobically fermented by bacteria, producing carbon dioxide, methane and hydrogen (hello, gas). For many, this process can cause irritation, gas and bloating. It can present as more severe if you are already suffering from sensitivities to FODMAPs or are battling with IBS. It is for this reason that we suggest avoiding cruciferous veggies in Stage 1 while your gut is healing. However, if you find that you can tolerate cruciferous vegetables, feel free to include them. Otherwise, we will reintroduce them once you have strengthened your digestive system.

NOTE I am a big fan of cruciferous vegetables and believe that many families don't eat enough of them. They are rich in glucoraphanin and myrosinase, which help create sulforaphane, which studies have shown helps protect against cancer. These very 'aromatic' veggies help promote our body's natural detoxification pathways and help protect our bodies from free radical damage and disease. They can be very beneficial for gut, skin and immune health. You just need to work on your gut health and sensitivity to them if you have one.

Avoid resistant starch (for now): Once your digestive system is feeling stronger and ready to be fed with more beneficial probiotics in Stage 3, we will introduce more resistant starch-containing foods. In Stage 1, however, when microbial imbalances in the small intestine are present we'll limit resistant starch to avoid any excessive fermentation in the gut.

Limit raw foods: These can be hard to digest and should be limited until your gut is feeling calmer. Once your gut is feeling strong again, raw veggies are an excellent source of nutrients, fibre and enzymes.

Limit nuts and seeds (for now): Nuts and seeds contain phytates that can impair digestion. If nuts don't irritate your gut, it's okay to keep them in. We recommend soaking, sprouting or activating them to assist in the breakdown of phytates.

NOTE If you are vegan and have limited sources of protein, you may need to continue eating nuts and seeds during Stage 1. To make them less irritating for your gut, try to include them in the form of activated nut and seed butter or finely ground, and remember to always soak them.

Limit gluten-free grains: Grains such as rice and gluten-free oats can be difficult for some people to digest. We will reintroduce them later in the Gut Guide as they are good sources of resistant starch. Grains also contain lectins, which can damage the gut lining and prevent proper absorption, which is why soaking them is so important.

Enjoy pseudo-grains such as quinoa and buckwheat (in moderation): They resemble grains, but are actually the seeds of grasses. The three major pseudo-grains are quinoa, buckwheat and amaranth, and they are superior to grains in several ways. Quinoa has a complete amino acid profile, while buckwheat and amaranth contain significant amounts of proteins. They all contain good levels of B vitamins and iron, making them great for those on a vegan diet.

NOTE Do not include a food that you have a known intolerance to or that upsets your gut, even if it is included in the Gut Guide. Some people report a sore and irritated gut when they eat quinoa, so only eat it if you tolerate it.

IMPORTANT FOODS & INGREDIENTS

ANTI-INFLAMMATORY FOODS

OMEGA-3 FATS: Found in walnuts, flaxseeds, chia seeds, wild salmon, trout, sardines and other cold water deep-sea fish.

BASIL: An anti-inflammatory herb. Studies show it may inhibit the same enzyme blocked by anti-inflammatory medications.

CALENDULA TEA: Used for its anti-inflammatory benefits in traditional herbal medicine.

DARK, LEAFY GREEN VEGETABLES: Rich in vitamins A, C, E and K, phytochemicals and chlorophyll, leafy greens are also rich in the antioxidant quercetin – a potent anti-inflammatory and great for healing the gut.

EXTRA-VIRGIN OLIVE OIL: Contains the anti-inflammatory compound oleocanthal.

FOODS RICH IN MAGNESIUM: Low magnesium may lead to inflammation, while higher levels help with constipation by relaxing the muscles of the intestinal wall. Magnesium is found in dark, leafy green and cruciferous veggies, avocado, legumes, seafood, cacao, bananas, seeds, tempeh and nuts. (NOTE: Some of these foods are not recommended for Stage 1.)

GINGER: Contains the powerful anti-inflammatory compound gingerol.

ROSEMARY: Its high flavonoid content makes it a potent anti-inflammatory.

TURMERIC: An anti-inflammatory spice that helps soothe an irritated digestive tract.

ALOE VERA: A rich source of vitamins, minerals, phytonutrients, fatty acids and enzymes. It is anti-inflammatory and may help soothe and ease the discomfort associated with gastrointestinal conditions.

BONE BROTH (PAGE 229): Bone broth is rich in glycine, an amino acid that the cells in our gut need to regenerate; proline, which helps support collagen production; and L-glutamine, which strengthens the intestinal barrier. Studies also show that amino acid-rich gelatin which is found in bone broth is excellent for healing and sealing the gut.

COD LIVER OIL: Rich in gut healing vitamin A, D and omega-3 fatty acids. Vitamin D deficiency has been linked to a decrease in the production of antimicrobial molecules essential for maintaining a healthy gut flora.

COLOSTRUM: The first form of milk produced by the mammary glands of mammals, immediately following the delivery of a newborn baby animal. Research shows that colostrum can help restore leaky gut lining to normal levels of permeability. Add 1 teaspoon to smoothies and porridges in the morning, if desired. Make sure that it is from grass-fed animals.

LICORICE ROOT: This adaptogenic herb helps heal leaky gut by activating anti-inflammatory pathways. Deglycyrrhizinated licorice (DGL) is a form of licorice root that can be taken long term.

MARSHMALLOW ROOT: A 2010 pre-clinical study found that the butyrate in marshmallow root can have a protective or therapeutic effect on inflammatory bowel diseases.

THE BEAUTY CHEF GUT PRIMER INNER BEAUTY SUPPORT: With L-glutamine, licorice root, slippery elm, aloe vera, zinc, turmeric, papaya and apple-cider vinegar. A complex formula designed to heal and seal your gut.

ORGANIC, GRASS-FED GHEE: Traditionally used in Ayurvedic medicine, ghee contains butyric acid, a powerful anti-inflammatory that has been linked to helping ulcerative colitis.

PARSLEY: Rich in quercetin, which in-vitro studies show can repair damage to the gut's mucosal lining.

PROTEIN-RICH FOODS: Protein breaks down into amino acids, which are the building blocks of our cells. The amino acid glutamine supports the repair of mucosal tissue and is found in many animal and plant-based proteins.

POLYPHENOLS: These antioxidant compounds are found in vegetables, fruits, nuts and seeds (carrots, celery, capsicum/bell pepper, sweet potato, spinach, broccoli, cabbage, green tea, black tea, cinnamon, cacao, peppermint, lemon, thyme, rosemary, capers, onions, garlic, ginger, tomatoes, pears, berries, linseeds/flaxseeds, quinoa, nuts, apples with skin on, pomegranate and olive oil). Animal studies show that they help improve gut barrier function (NOTE: not all of these foods are recommended in Stage 1).

SLIPPERY ELM POWDER: A mucilage powder used to soothe the entire digestive tract and help to repair the gut's mucosal layer.

ZINC-RICH FOODS: Zinc is necessary in maintaining intestinal wall integrity, and studies show that a deficiency of zinc may have a significant effect on the microbial population and diversity in the gut. Shellfish (not included in the Gut Guide), red meat, chicken, legumes, cacao and eggs are all good sources of zinc. Pumpkin seeds (pepitas), yoghurt and kefir are also good sources, while spinach, beans and kale are okay ones (NOTE: Not all of these foods are recommended in Stage 1).

VITAMIN D-RICH FOODS: Found in salmon, sardines, egg yolks and mushrooms, vitamin D can help heal the gut wall, while a deficiency has an adverse effect on the microbiome. (NOTE: Mushrooms are a great source of nutrients, but because of the likelihood of mould they should only be eaten post-Gut Guide.)

VITAMIN A-RICH FOODS: Vitamin A is found in cod liver oil, liver and eggs; pro-vitamin A is found in leafy greens and orange and yellow veggies. Vitamin A helps support the integrity of the mucosal membrane and the immune system.

L-GLUTAMINE: A gut-healing amino acid found in foods including bone broth, grass fed meat, fish, turkey, asparagus, cabbage, spirulina and broccoli. While not all of these foods are recommended in Stage 1 of the Gut Guide, L-glutamine in its supplement form is an excellent support for leaky gut.

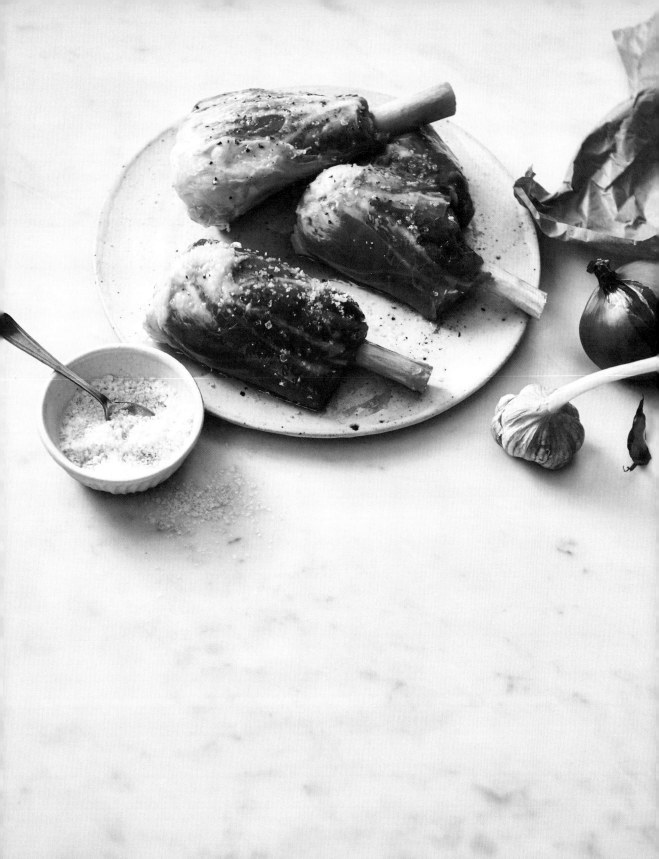

Stage 1 Meal Plan Options

* This recipe belongs in a later stage in its unadulterated form, but is suitable for Stage 1 with the suggested changes.

Stage 1 Sample Meal Plan

This chart offers an example of how you might build a meal plan for the healing stage. Remember, this stage is meant to be simple so that your gut can heal and strengthen.

A great way to prepare for the weeks ahead, and ensure you stay on track in every stage, is to prepare some of the elements from each recipe ahead of time. Plan your menu and do your grocery shop for the whole week's worth of meals. Or, if you have limited fridge space, prepare your shopping lists for the first few days and repeat midweek. Make big batches of the basics and freeze them, and use leftovers from dinner the night before as lunch the next day. These tricks save a lot of time and waste, and are a great way to stay organised.

	Upon Waking	Breakfast	Lunch	Snack (optional)	Dinner
M	2 tsp apple-cider vinegar or lemon juice in 125 ml (4 fl oz/½ cup) warm water ½ hour before first meal	2 slices Low-FODMAP Charcoal Flatbread, Zucchini Gremolata Dip & 2 poached eggs	Fennel & Chive Noodle Soup	Toasted Togarashi Nori Chips, without sesame seeds	Spiced Chicken, Three Ways with Gut-Healing Turmeric & Parsley Tabouleh
T	1 shot Bone Broth or Vegetarian Broth	Calming Smoothie	Pick-Your-Own-Herbs Oven-Baked Barramundi & Carrot Noodles	Raspberry, Licorice & Star Anise Gummies	Vegetable, Tapenade & Béchamel Bake with Green Beans, Sautéed Fennel, Capers & Herbs
W	2 tsp apple-cider vinegar or lemon juice in 125 ml (4 fl oz/½ cup) warm water ½ hour before first meal	2 slices Low-FODMAP Charcoal Flatbread, Nut-free Romesco & 2 poached eggs	Fennel & Chive Noodle Soup	Raspberry Mousse	Spiced Middle Eastern Lamb Koftas, low-FODMAP version
T	1 shot Bone Broth or Vegetarian Broth	Calming Smoothie	Buckwheat Pasta tossed with Nut-Free Roasted Romesco	Toasted Togarashi Nori Chips, without sesame seeds	Lemongrass & Kaffir Lime Salmon Cakes, without slaw
F	2 tsp apple-cider vinegar or lemon juice in 125 ml (4 fl oz/½ cup) warm water ½ hour before first meal	Herbed & Spiced Turmeric Eggs	Spiced Carrot & Tempeh Fritters	Papaya with Lime Yoghurt & Toasted Coconut	Baked Yoghurt & Herb Salmon with Fennel & Lemon, without yoghurt & pine nuts
S	1 shot Bone Broth or Vegetarian Broth	Romesco Baked Eggs	Spiced Barramundi & Masala Fried 'Rice', low-FODMAP version	Raspberry, Licorice & Star Anise Gummies	Spiced Chicken, Three Ways with Green Beans, Sautéed Fennel, Capers & Herbs
S	1 shot Bone Broth or Vegetarian Broth	Stracciatella Savoury Breakfast Soup	Spiced Middle Eastern Lamb Koftas, low-FODMAP version	Papaya with Lime Yoghurt & Toasted Coconut	Tangy Tempeh Green Curry

Stage 2: Weed

2 Weeks

Now that we have spent the last few weeks calming and healing the gut, the next two weeks will focus on helping to eliminate unwanted pathogens by incorporating antifungal and anti-parasitic foods. Think of your gut as a garden. If the garden is overrun with weeds (the bacteria we don't want), you would first need to remove the weeds and nurture the soil (your gut) before planting any seeds (the bacteria we do want). If the soil is unhealthy, the seeds won't sprout, and if they do they may not grow to their full potential.

For the remainder of the Gut Guide, we will continue to exclude any processed foods, along with refined sugars, gluten and unfermented and cows' dairy to help avoid inflammation and digestive disturbance. We also keep natural fruit sugars to a minimum until the gut heals.

IMPORTANT FOODS & INGREDIENTS

FOODS THAT STIMULATE AND IMPROVE DIGESTION

Improving your ability to break down and absorb nutrients is very important when healing and soothing the gut wall. Almost all digestive problems can be traced back to compromised digestive function. Below are a number of ways to boost digestive enzymes and acids. Some people will use supplemental enzymes (I recommend using them under a practitioner's guidance), but why not try and stimulate with herbs and foods first?

BITTER FOODS: They stimulate bile flow from the liver, promoting healthy fat digestion (rocket/arugula, dandelion greens, chard, kale, spinach, chicory, endive, artichoke, broccoli and cabbage).

BITTER HERBS: They include globe artichoke, St Mary's thistle, dandelion root and Oregon grape root.

CLEANSING AND ALKALISING FOODS: Green leafy vegetables, lemon, avocado, apple-cider vinegar and liquid chlorophyll.

MILK THISTLE: Stimulates bile production for healthy fat digestion.

PEPPERMINT: Has a relaxant effect on the gut muscles, which helps digestive function.

SOUR FOODS: Contain enzymes that help break down food (lemon, lime, tomato, tamarind, yoghurt and apple-cider vinegar).

SWEDISH BITTERS: Research has shown that bitters act on tastebud receptors to stimulate the secretion of saliva in the mouth and hydrochloric acid in the stomach.

UNPASTEURISED APPLE-CIDER VINEGAR: When taken just before a meal, it acts as a natural digestive stimulant and improves the breakdown of food.

ZINC-RICH FOODS: Animal studies show that zinc deficiency reduces digestive enzymes, so boost your consumption of zinc-rich foods. Shellfish (not included in the Gut Guide), red meat, chicken, legumes, pumpkin seeds (pepitas), cacao and eggs are good sources of zinc. Goat and sheep's yoghurt are also good sources, but not for Stage 2 of the guide. Spinach, beans and kale are okay sources.

NATURAL ANTI-INFLAMMATORY, ANTIFUNGAL AND ANTI-PARASITIC FOODS

CORIANDER SEEDS: A natural anti-inflammatory and antispasmodic that relaxes the muscles in the gastrointestinal tract.

CUMIN: It is anti-inflammatory and may help relieve symptoms associated with irritable bowel syndrome.

EXTRA-VIRGIN COCONUT OIL: Rich in antifungal lauric acid and caprylic acid.

GARLIC: Contains the active ingredient allicin, which helps fight candida, pathogenic bacteria and parasites. It is thought to spare the beneficial bacteria, unlike synthetic antibiotics.

GINGER: Contains gingerol, which may destroy parasites including roundworm, blood fluke, anisakis worm and salmonella bacteria.

NUTMEG: Promotes antifungal activity against pathogenic fungi. Use in moderation.

ONIONS: Contain sulphur compounds with strong antifungal and anti-parasitic properties.

OREGANO: An anti-parasitic. Incorporate into your diet both fresh and dried.

POLYPHENOLS: The antioxidant compounds found in vegetables, fruits, nuts and seeds support the inhibition of pathogenic bacteria and yeast overgrowth.

PUMPKIN SEEDS (PEPITAS): They contain natural anti-parasitic properties that may help fight against intestinal worms.

THYME: Contains flavonoids known as thymol and carvacrol, which fight against certain bacteria and fungal/yeast infections.

TURMERIC: Anti-inflammatory, antiseptic and antibacterial.

ANTI-PARASITIC NUTRIENTS AND HERBS

These potent ingredients are often included in herbal anti-parasitic formulas. These compounds shouldn't be used for prolonged periods and must be taken under the care of a practitioner, as they need to be rotated and checked for safety and effectiveness.

BLACK WALNUT: Works well as an anti-parasitic.

CLOVE OIL: Traditionally used to treat parasite eggs, *Candida albicans*, *Staphylococcus* and *Escherichia coli*.

GRAPESEED EXTRACT: Use with caution, as it is non-selective and will destroy beneficial bacteria as well as the pathogenic kind.

OREGANO OIL: High in phenols, which make it a powerful anti-parasitic and antifungal.

PHELLODENDRON: Contains berberine, used in traditional Chinese medicine to maintain digestive health in the small intestine.

THYME OIL: An effective antifungal and antibacterial agent with the ability to destroy worms.

WORMWOOD: Effective against bacteria and intestinal worms.

NOTE If you have been diagnosed with a parasite or bacterial infection (common strains include, but are not limited to, *Dientamoeba fragilis*, *Blastocystis hominis* or *Helicobacter pylori*), then you need to consult with a practitioner to discuss treatment options. Often a treatment regime will need to include pharmaceutical antibiotics along with herbal antimicrobials to get the best result.

Stage 2 Meal Plan Options

Feel free to also include any recipes from Stage 1 in your meal plan.

Stage 2 Sample Meal Plan

Here is a sample of what a week on Stage 2 might look like. Soups are a great source of nutrients while also being gentle on digestion. As Stage 2 is all about weeding, boosting your digestive enzymes and continuing the healing process, we have focused primarily on soups, limited red meat intake and removed foods known to cause inflammation.

	Upon Waking	Breakfast	Lunch	Snack (optional)	Dinner
M	Jamu Tonic	Papaya Cleanse Smoothie	Fennel & Chive Noodle Soup (page 186)	Buckwheat & Caraway Crackers with Garlicky Hummus	Fig, Garlic & Oregano Braised Chicken with steamed green beans
T	Umeboshi, Lemon, Ginger & Manuka Honey Tonic	Spiced Pear Porridge	Zucchini, Fennel, Mint & Basil Soup	Peppermint & Cacao Tea	Grilled Sardines on Fried Buckwheat Cakes with Silverbeet & Harissa
W	Jamu Tonic	2 slices Low-FODMAP Charcoal Flatbread (page 235), Nut-Free Roasted Romesco (page 241) & 2 poached eggs	Okra, Roasted Tomato & Buckwheat Noodle Bowl with Miso Ginger Broth	Toasted Togarashi Nori Chips	Herb-Infused Chicken Patties & Green Beans with Miso, Tahini & Umeboshi Dressing
T	Umeboshi, Lemon, Ginger & Manuka Honey Tonic	Spiced Pear Porridge	Buckwheat Pasta (page 233) with Nut-Free Roasted Romesco (page 241)	Peppermint & Cacao Tea	Tamarind Fish Curry with Turmeric Roti
F	Jamu Tonic	Papaya Cleanse Smoothie	Parsnip, Leek & Apple Soup with Walnut Dukkah	Buckwheat & Caraway Crackers with Zucchini Gremolata Dip (page 205)	Chicken, Vegetable & Buckwheat Soup
S	Jamu Tonic	Romesco Baked Eggs (page 109)	Beet & Daikon Soup with Rocket Pesto	Passionfruit Panna Cotta	Spiced Middle Eastern Lamb Koftas with Gut-Healing Turmeric & Parsley Tabouleh (page 198)
S	Jamu Tonic	Sweet Potato, Miso & Buckwheat Porridge	Harira Lamb Shank Soup	Papaya with Lime Yoghurt & Toasted Coconut (page 210)	Dill-Infused Fish, Leek & Spinach Soup

Stage 3: Seed

2 Weeks

As well as following the guidelines outlined in Stage 2, Stage 3 is where we plant the seeds for good gut health, focussing on foods that help implant beneficial bacteria into your gut and promote microbial diversity. These include probiotic-rich foods like fermented vegetables and coconut kefir. Probiotics are live bacteria that help to keep your digestive system happy and healthy, and, like all organisms, they need sustenance to survive. With this in mind, we will also introduce small amounts of prebiotic-rich foods. These are non-digestible fibres that pass through the small intestine (that's right, undigested!) straight into the colon, providing the perfect source of nutrition for the bacteria we want more of. These prebiotic fibres also promote the production of short-chain fatty acids, reducing the mucosal interaction of intestinal pathogens (the bacteria we don't want). Introduce moderate amounts of these in Stage 3. By the time you get to Stage 4, you can introduce a lot more into your daily diet if you tolerate them.

Start by adding small amounts of fermented vegetables and foods, as they contain probiotics and prebiotics that will feed the beneficial bacteria in your gut. We also increase the amount of nuts and seeds at this stage. But be sure that your system is ready. If any of these foods cause a lot of bloating and discomfort, then reduce them and go slower when reintroducing them.

Most health food stores and even supermarkets now sell fermented foods, such as sauerkraut, kefir and kimchi. If you would like to learn more about the art and science of fermentation, there is a whole chapter on it in *The Beauty Chef Cookbook*.

This is a great time to introduce The Beauty Chef's prebiotic, probiotic and postbiotic powders and elixirs, but of course they are optional.

IMPORTANT FOODS & INGREDIENTS

PREBIOTIC & PROBIOTIC FOODS

FERMENTED FOODS: Rich in bioactive molecules and probiotics, which are an important part of your gut-healing journey. Some of my favourites are miso, kimchi, sauerkraut, coconut kefir, natto and tempeh.

POLYPHENOLS: Not only are polyphenols integral in terms of healing the gut, they also encourage the growth of beneficial bacteria, promoting microbial diversity.

PREBIOTIC-RICH FOODS: Jerusalem artichoke, bananas, asparagus, onions, garlic, cabbage, beans, legumes, leeks, root vegetables and apples (skin on).

Stage 3 Meal Plan Options

Breakfast

Nourish Smoothie	95
Kimchi, Avocado & Spinach Omelette	108
Coconut Crêpes with Coconut Yoghurt & Berries	111

Lunch & Dinner

Salmon Lunch Bowl	117
Baked Yoghurt & Herb Salmon with Fennel & Lemon	118
Kingfish Ceviche, Spiced Coconut & Tamarind Egg Bowl	128
Saffron Fish Chowder	132
Chicken, Wombok, Asparagus & Pea Soup	137
Baked Lemon Chicken with Leeks & Green Olives	140
Vietnamese-Style Chicken Lettuce Cups	145
Swedish Meatballs with Braised Red Cabbage	149
Cauliflower & Tempeh Falafel with Tahini Sauce	168
Lentil Moussaka	173
Ginger & Miso Sweet Potato Soup with Wakame	177
Roasted Jerusalem Artichoke Soup	182

Sides & Snacks

Sweet Potato Chips with Lime Cream	190
Spice-Roasted Cauliflower with Nut Butter Cream, Almonds & Herbs	195
Broccoli & Asparagus Tabouleh	200
Baked Postbiotic Kimchi	202
Zucchini, Apple, Walnut & Cardamom Loaf	209

Desserts

Raw Blueberry, Lavender & Coconut Cream Flan	220

Basics

Kimchi with Daikon, Cabbage & Apple	230
Sauerkraut with Carrot, Caraway Seeds & Juniper Berries	236
Prebiotic Superseed Bread	242
Pumpkin Seed & Herb Pesto	244
Probiotic Butter, Two Ways	245

Feel free to also include any recipes from Stages 1 & 2 in your meal plan.

Stage 3 Sample Meal Plan

Here is a sample of what a week on Stage 3 might look like, with a focus on incorporating probiotic-rich foods to seed the gut.

	Upon Waking	Breakfast	Lunch	Snack (optional)	Dinner
M	Jamu Tonic (page 84)	Nourish Smoothie	Ginger & Miso Sweet Potato Soup with Wakame	1 slice Prebiotic Superseed Bread with Pumpkin Seed & Herb Pesto & Sauerkraut	Swedish Meatballs with Braised Red Cabbage
T	Peppermint & Cacao Tea (page 88)	Kimchi, Avocado & Spinach Omelette	Roasted Jerusalem Artichoke Soup	Papaya with Lime Yoghurt & Toasted Coconut (page 210)	Lentil Moussaka with Green Beans, Sautéed Fennel, Capers & Herbs (page 199)
W	Jamu Tonic (page 84)	Sweet Potato, Miso & Buckwheat Porridge (page 101)	Salmon Lunch Bowl	Toasted Togarashi Nori Chips (page 210)	Chicken, Wombok, Asparagus & Pea Soup
T	Peppermint & Cacao Tea (page 88)	Nourish Smoothie	Vietnamese-Style Chicken Lettuce Cups	1 slice Prebiotic Superseed Bread with Pumpkin Seed & Herb Pesto & Sauerkraut	Saffron Fish Chowder
F	Jamu Tonic (page 84)	Herbed & Spiced Turmeric Eggs (page 103)	Spiced Carrot & Tempeh Fritters (page 176)	Zucchini, Apple, Walnut & Cardamom Loaf	Baked Yoghurt & Herb Salmon with Fennel & Lemon
S	Peppermint & Cacao Tea (page 88)	Coconut Crêpes with Coconut Yoghurt & Berries	Kingfish Ceviche, Spiced Coconut & Tamarind Egg Bowl	Toasted Togarashi Nori Chips (page 210)	Baked Lemon Chicken with Leek & Green Olives with Spice-Roasted Cauliflower with Nut Butter Cream, Almonds & Herbs
S	Peppermint & Cacao Tea (page 88)	Stracciatella Savoury Breakfast Soup (page 106)	Cauliflower & Tempeh Falafel with Tahini Sauce with Broccoli & Asparagus Tabouleh	Papaya with Lime Yoghurt & Toasted Coconut (page 210)	Herb-Infused Chicken Patties (page 141) with Sweet Potato Chips with Lime Cream

Stage 4: Feed

2 Weeks

The final stage of the program focuses on 'feeding' the gut by providing fuel (prebiotics) for the beneficial bacteria (probiotics) that we have planted. Here, we introduce more fibre and resistant starch, which are very important when it comes to feeding the beneficial bacteria in our gut, keeping the gut cells healthy and resilient. We also increase consumption of nuts, seeds and raw foods.

IMPORTANT FOODS & INGREDIENTS

HIGH-FIBRE FOODS

Foods that contain both soluble and insoluble fibre promote regular bowel motions, which is important when reducing unfriendly yeasts and bacteria in the gut.

HERBS AND SPICES

LEGUMES
(soaking is recommended, see page 57)

VEGETABLES AND FRUITS
(listed in 'Enjoy' and 'Foods only allowed at certain stages of the Gut Guide' columns, page 53)

RAW FOODS, SEEDS AND NUTS
(I recommend soaking the nuts, see page 57)

RESISTANT STARCH

By Stage 4, you can start adding more resistant starch into your diet to help feed your friendly microbes. Resistant starch is extremely beneficial for digestive health as its fermentation helps produce butyrate, which improves the gut's integrity. When introducing resistant starches into your diet, go slow and only eat them in moderation. The below foods can be used to create your own recipes or used as substitutes for recipes in the Gut Guide (swapping cauliflower rice for cooked and cooled white basmati rice, for example). Resistant starch can cause bloating, so take it slowly!

RICE: When rice is cooked, cooled and reheated, the levels of resistant starch are increased and the glycaemic index is lowered. We recommend eating rice in moderation and opting for white basmati rice as it is low GI and easier to digest than brown rice, especially while healing your gut. Be mindful of appropriate handling and storage to avoid botulism contamination. Store cooked rice in the refrigerator and consume within 3 days.
(For cooking and soaking methods, see page 57).

GREEN BANANAS AND PLANTAINS

GREEN BANANA FLOUR

WHITE POTATOES: Make sure to boil and then cool potatoes before mashing or roasting them – it increases levels of resistant starch and lowers the GI. Because the GI is still relatively high, eat them in moderation. Nicola and Carisma potatoes have a lower GI.

POTATO STARCH: Add up to 1 tablespoon to your smoothies or yoghurt.

COOKED AND COOLED LEGUMES

GLUTEN-FREE OATS: Only if tolerated. Remember to soak them to help improve their digestibility.

NOTE If supplementing with potato starch or green banana flour, start with very small doses: about 1 teaspoon once a day, and gradually increase as they are tolerated. Studies show the benefits of resistant starch in relation to insulin sensitivity manifest when consuming 15 to 30 grams (½ to 1 oz) daily.

Stage 4 Meal Plan Options

The Beauty Chef Gut Guide

Feel free to also include any recipes from Stages 1, 2 & 3 in your meal plan.

Stage 4 Sample Meal Plan

Here is a sample of what a week in Stage 4 might look like. Building on the principles from Stages 2 & 3, we introduce more foods rich in prebiotics, fibre and resistant starch to further promote microbial diversity and a healthy belly. Again, planning your meals for the weeks ahead is a great way to stay organised and on track.

	Upon Waking	Breakfast	Lunch	Snack (optional)	Dinner
M	Slow-Pressed Green Juice with Aloe Vera & Chia	Kimchi, Avocado & Spinach Omelette (page 108)	Indian-Spiced Sweet Potato & Lentil Cakes	1 slice Prebiotic Superseed Bread (page 242) with Pumpkin Seed & Herb Pesto (page 244) & Sauerkraut (page 236)	Chicken Katsu Don
T	Umeboshi, Lemon, Ginger & Manuka Honey Tonic (page 88)	Coconut Crêpes with Coconut Yoghurt & Berries (page 111)	Spiced Middle Eastern Lamb Koftas (page 152) with Roasted Carrot, Witlof & Toasted Walnut Salad with Orange & Umeboshi Dressing	Artichoke & Green Olive Dip with carrot & celery sticks	Pick-Your-Own-Herbs Oven-Baked Barramundi (page 134) with Baked Postbiotic Kimchi (page 202)
W	Slow-Pressed Green Juice with Aloe Vera & Chia	Sautéed Silverbeet, Sheep's Yoghurt & Poached Eggs	Spiced Barramundi & Masala Fried 'Rice'	Toasted Togarashi Nori Chips (page 210)	Chicken, Vegetable & Buckwheat Soup (page 136)
T	Umeboshi, Lemon, Ginger & Manuka Honey Tonic (page 88)	Glowing Gut Smoothie	Pick-Your-Own-Herbs Oven-Baked Barramundi (page 134) with Miso, Potato & Eggplant Salad	Artichoke & Green Olive Dip with carrot & celery sticks	Chicken, Flaked Almond & Sage Buckwheat 'Risotto'
F	Slow-Pressed Green Juice with Aloe Vera & Chia	Sri Lankan Scrambled Eggs with Coconut Sambol	Lemongrass & Kaffir Lime Salmon Cakes	Hazelnut, Apricot & Cacao Nib Cookies with Peppermint & Cacao Tea (page 88)	Pan-Fried Cauliflower Gnocchi with Creamy Pesto
S	Dandelion Chai	Banana, Coconut & Turmeric Muffins	Spring Tart with Asparagus, Peas & Herbs	Artichoke & Green Olive Dip with carrot & celery sticks	Anise-Roasted Pumpkin Agnolotti with Walnuts, Sage & Browned Butter
S	Dandelion Chai	Vanilla & Cardamom Chia Pudding	Slow-Cooked Beef Cheek with Onions & Raisins	Papaya with Coconut Lime Yoghurt & Toasted Coconut (page 210)	Beet & Daikon Soup with Rocket Pesto (page 181)

Post-Gut Guide Protocol

Once you have completed the four stages of the Gut Guide, continue to use the recipes and guidelines from this book to maintain a balanced, gut-friendly diet. Your gut has been strengthened and nourished with the prebiotics and probiotics it needs to help maintain a healthy microbiota, so you will be able to reintroduce and include other foods sporadically that aren't included in the program. The key is to listen to your gut as it will tell you whether it agrees with what you are feeding it.

SUGGESTIONS FOR LIFE BEYOND THE GUT GUIDE

1 If you are reintroducing gluten-containing foods, try to make smart choices. For example, eat organic sourdough or spelt bread instead of white sliced bread.

2 While remaining dairy free is recommended, as it is inflammatory for many people, you can add more fermented dairy (goats and sheeps' yoghurt and cheese, for example).

3 Reintroduce foods that you can tolerate in small amounts.

4 Add small amounts of resistant starch (such as cooked and cooled white basmati rice and potatoes).

5 Small amounts of red wine can be enjoyed occasionally and in moderation. Red wine is rich in antioxidants known as polyphenols, which help to protect the lining of blood vessels in the heart.

6 Drink coffee and tea in moderation.

7 Avoid processed packet foods and refined sugars.

8 Enjoy fruit sugars and natural sweeteners such as honey and pure organic maple syrup in moderation.

9 Eat lots of types of vegetables, good amounts of healthy fats, legumes, nuts, seeds and fruits alongside smaller amounts of good-quality animal protein. Think Mediterranean diet.

10 Eat certified organic foods wherever possible.

11 Drink lots of filtered water daily.

12 Continue to work with your health practitioner.

13 Eat raw vegetables if your gut is feeling robust, as they are rich in enzymes. However, if your tummy is sensitive, lightly steam them or put them in nutrient-rich soups instead.

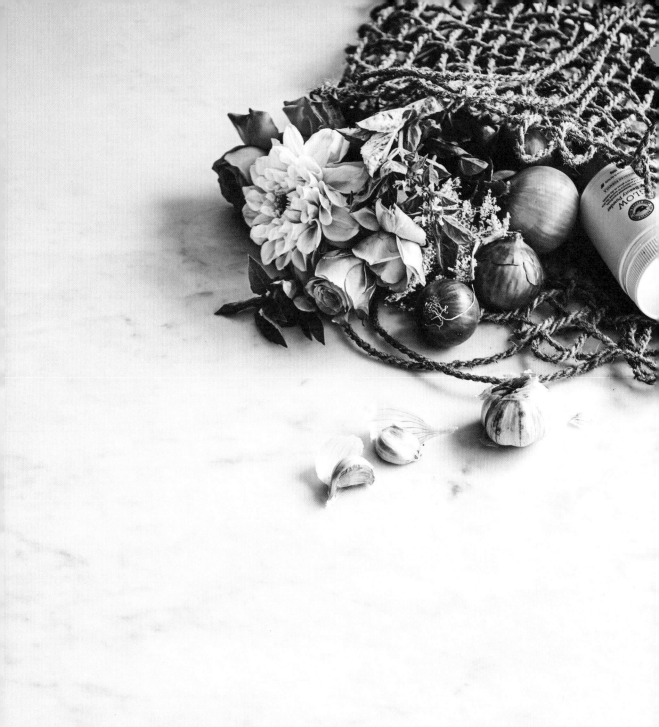

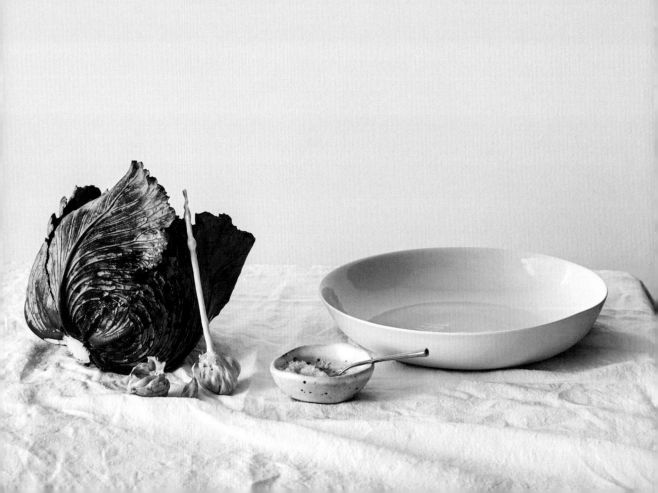

Part 3

Recipes

Dietary Tag Index

Gluten Free   Strictly excludes gluten or gluten-containing products.

Dairy Free   Strictly excludes dairy or dairy-containing products (except for those listed in the 'Enjoy' column on page 55).

Dairy-Free Option   Alternative suggestions are given so you can make the recipe dairy free.

NOTE: Although ghee is technically dairy and we treat it as such, it contains almost no casein or lactose and is considered beneficial for your gut.

Vegetarian   Strictly excludes all meat and fish. Includes eggs and dairy listed in the 'Enjoy freely' column (page 55).

Vegetarian Option   Alternative ingredient suggestions are given so you can make the recipe vegetarian. Includes eggs and dairy listed in the 'Enjoy freely' column (page 55).

Vegan   Strictly excludes all meat, fish and animal-derived products such as eggs, dairy and honey.

Vegan Option   Alternative ingredient suggestions are given so you can make the recipe vegan.

Low FODMAP   Does not contain any foods classified as high FODMAP according to the Monash University low-FODMAP diet guidelines.

NOTE: Many recipes not marked with this label can be adapted to be low FODMAP: just look for a note at the bottom labeled as 'Low-FODMAP Option'. Please also note that these recipes are classified as low FODMAP at one serve per person only. Please be aware that an increase in serving size may alter the level of FODMAPs in a given recipe.

Stage 1 Friendly   Recipes suitable for introducing in Stage 1 of the Gut Guide, which can also be used throughout Stages 2, 3 & 4.

Stage 2 Friendly   Recipes suitable for introducing in Stage 2 of the Gut Guide, which can also be used throughout Stages 3 & 4.

Stage 3 Friendly   Recipes suitable for introducing in Stage 3 of the Gut Guide, which can also be used throughout Stage 4.

Stage 4 Friendly   Recipes suitable for introducing in Stage 4 of the Gut Guide.

This book uses metric cup measurements, i.e. 250 ml for 1 cup; in the US a cup is 8 fl oz, just smaller, and American cooks should be generous in their cup measurements; in the UK a cup is 10 fl oz and British cooks should be scant with their cup measurements. This book uses 20 ml (¾ fl oz) tablespoons; cooks with 15 ml (½ fl oz) tablespoons need to adjust accordingly.

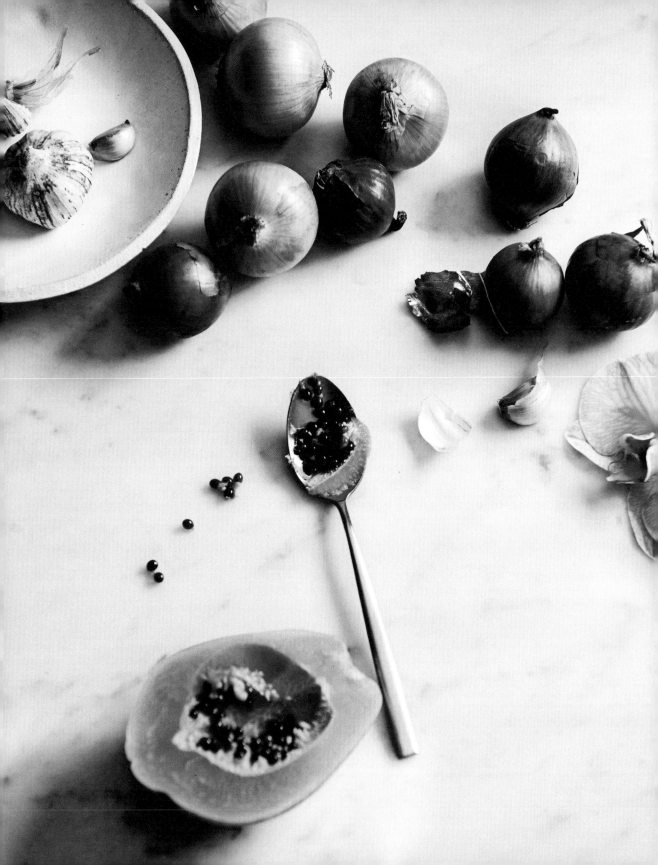

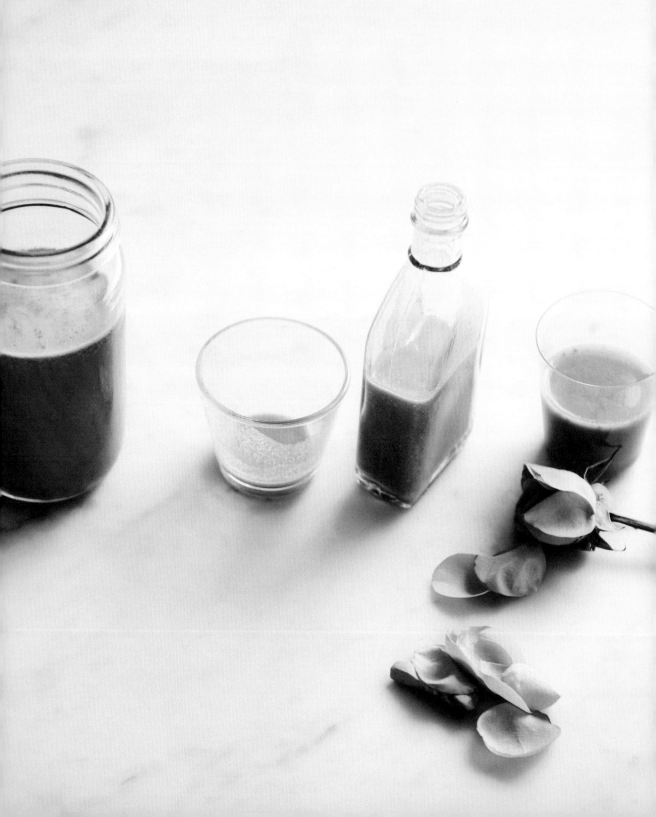

Tonics & Healing Elixirs

Jamu Tonic

Jamu is an Indonesian herbal drink traditionally used for medicinal healing. Sweet-and-sour tamarind, ginger and spicy turmeric are a powerful combination when it comes to fighting inflammation and supporting digestive health. Manuka honey provides a little more than just sweetness, with natural antibiotic qualities that make it great for bacteria-related issues and gastrointestinal imbalances.

SERVES 8 (Makes approx. 1 litre/34 fl oz/4 cups)

1 cinnamon stick, broken into pieces

¼ teaspoon black peppercorns

1 litre (34 fl oz/4 cups) water

2 tablespoons fresh ginger, finely chopped

juice & zest of 1 unwaxed lime

250 ml (8½ fl oz/1 cup) tinned coconut milk

85 g (3 oz/⅓ cup) seedless tamarind purée

3 tablespoons ground turmeric

80 ml (2½ fl oz/⅓ cup) active honey,
     such as manuka or Jellybush

In a medium saucepan, toast the cinnamon and peppercorns over a low–medium heat for 30 seconds, or until fragrant. Pour in the water, then add the ginger and lime zest and bring to the boil. Reduce to a simmer for 5 minutes, then set aside until cooled to room temperature.

Add the lime juice, coconut milk, tamarind, turmeric and honey and stir to combine. Strain the tonic through a fine-mesh sieve, then pour into a sterilised 1 litre (34 fl oz) glass bottle or jar. Seal and store in the refrigerator for up to 2 weeks. Alternatively, pour into ice cube trays and freeze to have on hand whenever desired. If necessary, before serving, gently warm the tonic to melt the coconut fat.

CARLA'S TIP I like to drink this tonic in the morning on an empty stomach, half an hour before breakfast.

LOW-FODMAP OPTION Reduce the turmeric to 2 tablespoons and swap the honey for pure organic maple syrup.

Gluten Free   Dairy Free   Vegetarian   Stage 2 Friendly   Low-FODMAP Option

Slow-Pressed Green Juice
with Aloe Vera & Chia

Being a good host to your microbiome means starting your day with a nutrient-balanced elixir that helps heal and seal your gut lining, stimulating the production of digestive enzymes and promoting the growth of beneficial bacteria. It may be asking a lot, but this juice does it all. It contains aloe vera, shown to aid digestion, regulate the stomach's pH balance and encourage healthy bowel movements.

SERVES 2 (Makes approx. 750 ml/25½ fl oz/3 cups)

250 ml (8½ fl oz/1 cup) coconut water

60 ml (2 fl oz/¼ cup) aloe vera juice

3 teaspoons chia seeds

6 large kale leaves, stems removed, roughly chopped

1 medium green apple, cored & roughly chopped

1 Lebanese (short) cucumber, chopped

100 g (3½ oz) broccoli stalks & or florets, roughly chopped

½ lemon, skin, pith & seeds removed, roughly chopped

4–6 cm (1½–2½ in) piece fresh ginger, roughly chopped

4 handfuls mint, leaves & stems

2 handfuls flat-leaf (Italian) parsley, leaves & stems

In a small bowl, combine the coconut water, aloe vera and chia seeds. Set aside for 10 minutes, or until the seeds hydrate and swell.

Pass the kale, apple, cucumber, broccoli, lemon, ginger and herbs through your juicer.

Add the coconut, aloe and chia mixture to the juice and stir well.

CARLA'S TIP The jury is still out as to whether or not cruciferous vegetables can significantly impact thyroid health, although they may in those deficient in selenium and iodine. If you are concerned, cooking them helps destroy some of their goitrogenic properties.

Gluten Free   Dairy Free   Vegetarian   Vegan   Stage 4 Friendly

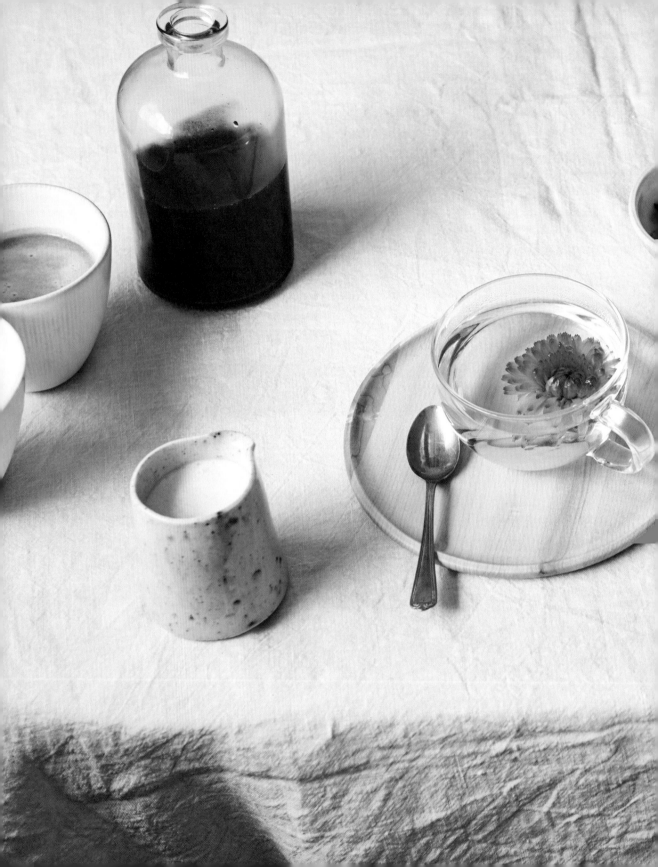

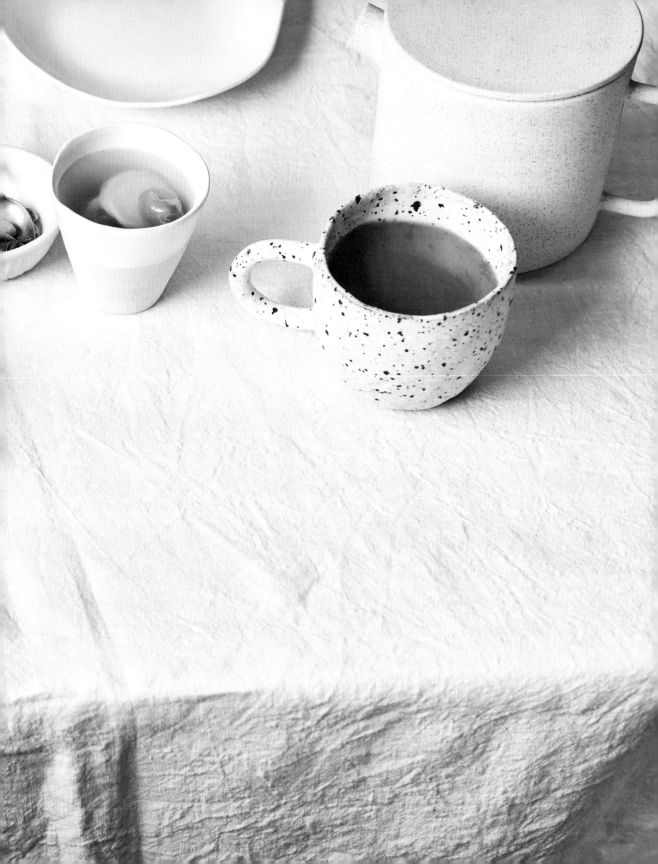

Umeboshi, Lemon, Ginger & Manuka Honey Tonic

Gluten Free   Dairy Free
Vegetarian   Stage 2 Friendly

This lovely tonic is ideal for Stage 2 of the Gut Guide. Ginger acts as a powerful anti-inflammatory, manuka honey brings potent anti-microbial benefits and studies show that consuming umeboshi plum daily helps to relieve reflux symptoms and improve gastric motility. Drink this upon waking, before your first meal of the day.

SERVES 1

1½ tablespoons freshly squeezed lemon juice
1 teaspoon manuka honey
1 cm (½ in) piece fresh ginger, thinly sliced
½ fermented umeboshi salted plum
250 ml (8½ fl oz/1 cup) just boiled water

Put all the ingredients in your favourite mug. Let steep for 3 minutes. Muddle the ingredients using a small teaspoon, sip and enjoy.

Image page 86/87

CARLA'S TIP You'll find umeboshi plums at most health food stores.

Peppermint & Cacao Tea

Gluten Free   Dairy Free
Vegetarian   Vegan
Stage 2 Friendly   Low FODMAP

Peppermint tea may be an age-old remedy for easing an unhappy gut, but science now confirms that the flavonoids in peppermint leaves, in particular hesperidin and luteolin, possess anti-inflammatory and analgesic qualities. With cacao acting as a helpful prebiotic for our gut flora, this warming cuppa is soothing, healing and great for sugar cravings too.

SERVES 1

1 peppermint tea bag
just boiled water
2 teaspoons raw cacao powder
½ teaspoon pure organic maple syrup, or to taste
1 teaspoon extra-virgin coconut oil
unsweetened UHT coconut, almond or macadamia milk, to taste

Put the tea bag in your favourite mug. Pour in enough boiled water to come three-quarters of the way up the sides of the mug and steep for 3–4 minutes, then discard the tea bag.

Add the cacao powder, maple syrup and coconut oil and stir to combine until the oil is melted. Top with some coconut milk and enjoy!

Image page 86/87

Dandelion Chai

Image page 87

Dandelion root is a natural, soothing digestive aid with a deep, nutty roasted flavour, making this brew a wonderful coffee replacement. Cinnamon, ginger and nutmeg add lots of aromatic spice as well as anti-inflammatory benefits to this delicious 'dandy chai'.

SERVES 1 (Makes enough syrup for 5, or 500 ml/17 fl oz/2 cups of chai)

100 ml (3½ fl oz) Dandy Chai Syrup
160 ml (5½ fl oz) drinking coconut, almond or macadamia milk

Dandy Chai Syrup
2 cinnamon sticks, broken
20 cardamom pods, bruised & opened
2 star anise
8 black peppercorns, cracked
4 whole cloves
5 cm (2 in) piece fresh ginger, sliced
1 teaspoon freshly grated nutmeg
2 litres (68 fl oz/8 cups) water
3 tablespoons roasted dandelion root
2 tablespoons manuka honey

To prepare the syrup, toast the cinnamon, cardamom, star anise, peppercorns and cloves in a small frying pan over a low heat for 30 seconds, or until fragrant.

Transfer the spices to a medium saucepan and add the ginger and nutmeg. Pour in the water, bring to the boil and boil for 45 minutes, or until reduced by approximately two-thirds. Add the dandelion root and simmer for 1 minute. Remove from the heat and set aside to steep for 10 minutes.

Strain the liquid through a fine-mesh sieve. Pour into a clean saucepan. Simmer for a further 15 minutes, or until reduced by approximately one-quarter, which should leave you with 500 ml (17 fl oz/2 cups) of syrup. If it reduces too much, add some water.

Remove the syrup from the heat, then add the honey and set aside to cool. Use immediately, transfer to an airtight container, or bottle and refrigerate until required. The syrup can be stored in the refrigerator for up to 1 month.

To make a cup of Dandelion Chai, combine 100 ml (3½ fl oz) of Dandy Chai Base with 160 ml (5½ fl oz) of your nut-based milk of choice in a small saucepan and bring to a simmer over a low heat for 3 minutes to reduce slightly and intensify the flavour. Pour into your favourite mug and enjoy!

CARLA'S TIP Cardamom is a wonderful digestive aid, making this drink perfect for before or after meals.

LOW-FODMAP OPTION Use unsweetened UHT coconut, almond or macadamia milk and swap the honey for some pure organic maple syrup.

Tonics & Healing Elixirs

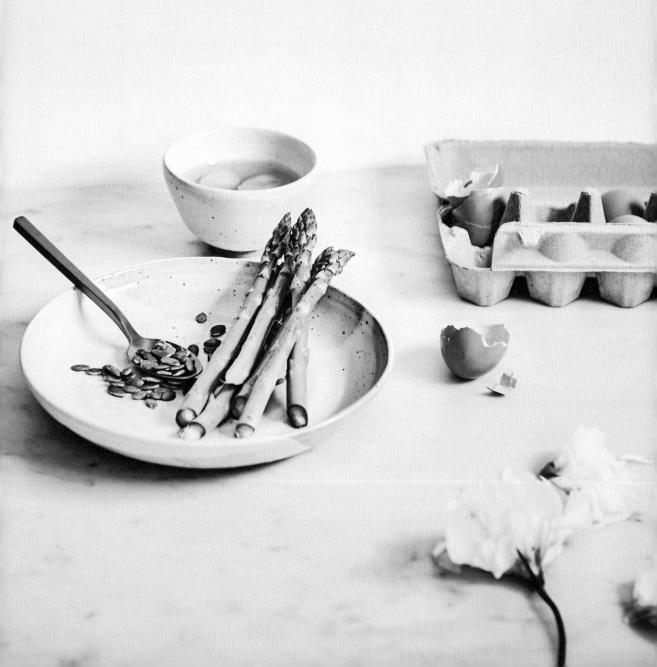

Breakfast

Calming Smoothie

Gluten Free
Vegetarian Option
Stage 1 Friendly

Dairy Free
Vegan Option
Low FODMAP

Stage 1 of the Gut Guide focuses on healing your digestive system, and this is the perfect restorative elixir. Slippery elm powder is a demulcent, acting as a barrier to soothe and protect the gut lining. Bone broth may sound like an unusual ingredient to add to a berry smoothie, but don't worry: the flavour flies under the radar, and your tummy will benefit from the calming and anti-inflammatory gelatin.

SERVES 2 (Makes approx. 750 ml/25½ fl oz/3 cups)

180 ml (6 fl oz/¾ cup) water
180 ml (6 fl oz/¾ cup) chilled beef Bone Broth or
    Vegetarian Broth (page 229), or store-bought stock
120 g (4½ oz/½ cup) frozen raspberries
60 g (2 oz/¼ cup) frozen blueberries
160 g (5½ oz/⅔ cup) coconut yoghurt
100 g (3½ oz /2 small) Lebanese (short) cucumber,
    roughly chopped
1 tablespoon slippery elm powder or The Beauty Chef
    Gut Primer Inner Beauty Support
2 teaspoons ground cinnamon
3 ice cubes

Combine all ingredients in a high-speed blender and blend until smooth.

CARLA'S TIP Coconut yoghurt has the tick of approval as FODMAP friendly as long as you keep it to 125 g (4½ oz/½ cup) per serve.

Glowing Gut Smoothie

Gluten Free
Vegetarian Option
Stage 4 Friendly

Dairy Free
Vegan Option

Chia seeds, once they've swelled, boast a smooth and satisfying texture rich with soothing mucilage gel. They contain a good mix of soluble and insoluble fibre that helps promote digestion, cleanse the system and keep you regular. This smoothie also has other fibre-rich ingredients, including berries, spinach, and green banana flour, which provides the resistant starch you need to help produce short-chain fatty acids such as butyrate, an anti-inflammatory important for keeping our gut lining healthy and our skin glowing.

SERVES 2 (Makes approx. 750 ml/25½ fl oz/3 cups)

180 ml (6 fl oz/¾ cup) chilled beef Bone Broth or
    Vegetarian Broth (page 229), or store-bought stock
120 g (4½ oz/1 cup) frozen mixed berries
    (blueberries, strawberries and/or raspberries)
1 medium ripe pear, roughly chopped
1 small banana
80 ml (2½ fl oz/⅓ cup) Coconut Milk Kefir (page 228)
    or coconut yoghurt
2 small handfuls baby spinach
1 tablespoon almond butter
2 teaspoons chia seeds
1 teaspoon green banana flour
2 teaspoons The Beauty Chef GLOW
    Inner Beauty Powder (optional)
3 ice cubes

Combine all ingredients in a high-speed blender and blend until smooth.

CARLA'S TIP You can find green banana flour at most health food stores and even some supermarkets. If you can't get your hands on it, swap for some potato starch: it's also a great source of resistant starch.

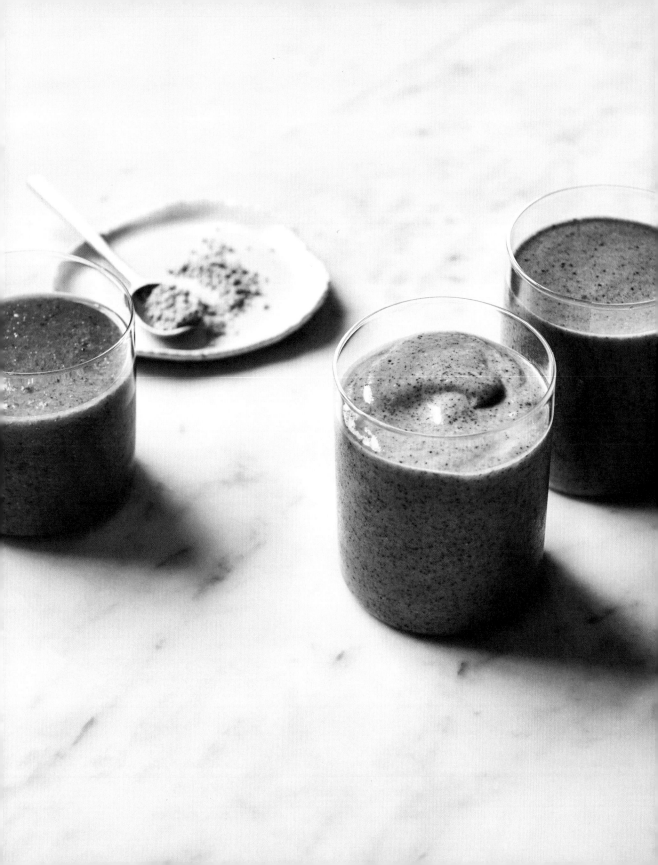

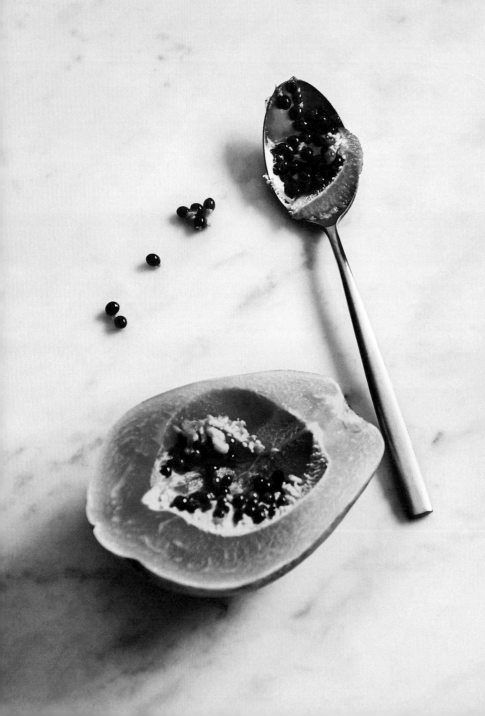

Papaya Cleanse Smoothie

Gluten Free
Vegetarian
Stage 2 Friendly

Dairy Free
Vegan Option
Low-FODMAP Option

Stage 2 of the Gut Guide focuses on detoxifying the body and introducing foods that help combat dysbiosis. Papaya is the perfect all-round gut-loving remedy. It's rich in papain, an enzyme that aids digestion by helping our bodies break down protein. Make sure to save the seeds – you'll be using them as well. A study showed that the anti-parasitic activity of these little seeds has a clearance rate of between 70 and 100 per cent when it comes to treating intestinal parasites.

SERVES 2 (Makes approx. 750 ml/25½ fl oz/3 cups)

270 g (9½ oz/1½ cups) red papaya
250 ml (8½ fl oz/1 cup) almond milk
90 g (3 oz/⅔ cup) frozen blackberries
125 ml (4 fl oz/½ cup) Coconut Milk Kefir (page 228)
    or coconut yoghurt
1 tablespoon freshly squeezed lime juice
1 tablespoon chia seeds
2 teaspoons papaya seeds (reserved from papaya)
2 teaspoons fresh ginger, finely chopped
1 teaspoon manuka honey (optional)
6 ice cubes

Combine all ingredients in a high-speed blender and blend until smooth.

CARLA'S TIP Coconut Milk Kefir is low FODMAP at 60 ml (2 fl oz/¼ cup) per serve.

LOW-FODMAP OPTION Swap blackberries for raspberries and omit the honey or use pure organic maple syrup in its place.

Nourish Smoothie

Gluten Free
Vegetarian
Stage 3 Friendly

Dairy Free
Vegan Option
Low-FODMAP Option

Stage 3 of the Gut Guide is all about repopulating the gut with beneficial bacteria, and coconut kefir is literally alive with it. This delicious, creamy drink helps inoculate your belly with a range of probiotics that help arm the gut against unfavourable bacteria while giving the immune system a boost. The selenium found in Brazil nuts acts as an anti-inflammatory, while avocado and blueberries offer good sources of polyphenols, fibre and healthy fats.

SERVES 2 (Makes approx. 750 ml/25½ fl oz/3 cups)

250 ml (8½ fl oz/1 cup) filtered or coconut water
125 ml (4 fl oz/½ cup) Coconut Milk Kefir (page 228)
    or coconut yoghurt
120 g (4½ oz/1 cup) frozen raspberries
1 medium green apple, cored & roughly chopped
½ medium avocado, stone removed
6 Brazil nuts
1 tablespoon freshly squeezed lemon juice
1 tablespoon chia seeds
1 teaspoon manuka honey (optional)
½ teaspoon ground cinnamon

Combine all ingredients in a high-speed blender and blend until smooth.

CARLA'S TIP Brazil nuts are a great source of selenium, a deficiency of which is associated with a higher risk of inflammatory bowel syndrome.

LOW-FODMAP OPTION Replace the apple with an unripe banana, the coconut water with almond milk, the avocado with half a cup of coconut yoghurt and the honey with pure organic maple syrup.

Vanilla & Cardamom Chia Puddings

The proof is in the pudding with this delicious, aromatic recipe. Chia provides 11 g (¼ oz) per serve of primarily soluble fibre, putting you well on your way to reaching your daily recommended intake and keeping your digestive tract happy (and moving). It's also rich in anti-inflammatory omega-3s. A hint of fragrant cardamom to aid digestion makes this super-easy breakfast soothing, yet satisfying. A scattering of blueberries will help boost your microbiome.

SERVES 2

180 ml (6 fl oz/¾ cup) water
8 cardamom pods, bruised with the side of a knife
310 ml (10½ fl oz/1¼ cups) drinking coconut or
    almond milk
60 g (2 oz/⅓ cup) chia seeds
1 teaspoon natural vanilla extract
stevia, to taste, or manuka honey (optional)
125 g (4½ oz/½ cup) coconut yoghurt, to serve
50 g (1¾ oz/⅓ cup) blueberries, blackberries
    or raspberries (whatever's in season), to serve
35 g (1¼ oz/¼ cup) pecans, roughly chopped, to serve

In a small saucepan, combine the water and cardamom pods and simmer for 5 minutes, or until the water is reduced by half. Add the coconut milk and bring back to a simmer. Remove the saucepan from the heat and set aside to infuse for 10 minutes.

Strain the infused milk through a sieve into a medium bowl. Add the chia seeds, vanilla and stevia and stir well to combine.

Pour the pudding into small jars or glasses and leave overnight for the seeds to swell and the pudding to thicken.

Serve the pudding with coconut yoghurt, berries and pecans.

CARLA'S TIP Make a double batch of chia puddings and store them in the refrigerator for up to 4 days to have on hand for a snack or quick dessert.

Gluten Free   Dairy Free   Vegetarian   Vegan Option   Stage 4 Friendly

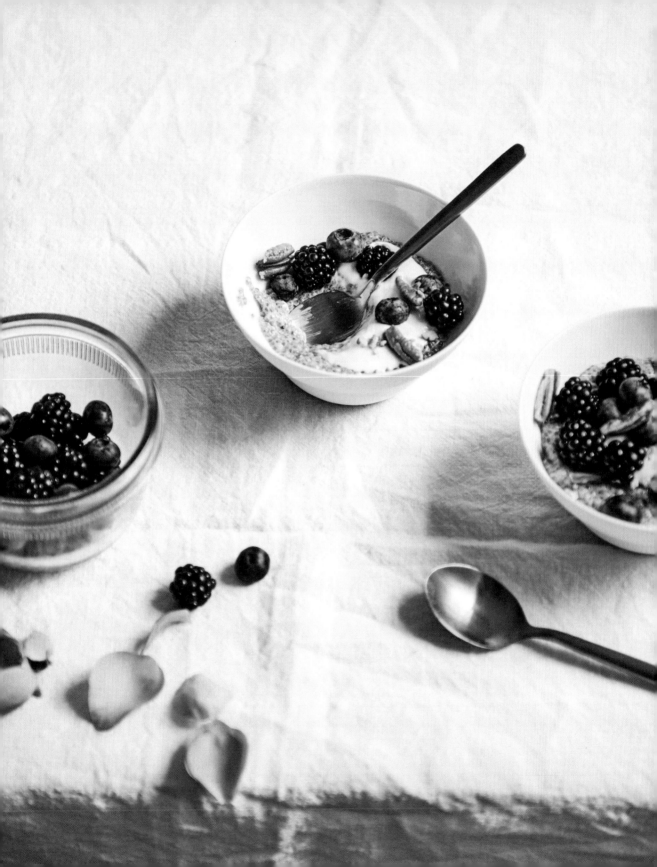

Spiced Pear Porridge

This delightfully spiced and nourishing porridge boasts all nine essential amino acids, which we need to obtain from food because our bodies can't make them. This porridge's lovely spices have anti-spasmodic and anti-fungal properties, and both pears and coconut milk bring anti-inflammatory benefits. They contain a prebiotic known as arabinogalactan, shown to stimulate the production of short-chain fatty acids – compounds that have a profound influence on the health of your microbiome, and therefore your health.

SERVES 2

125 ml (4 fl oz/½ cup) water
500 ml (17 fl oz/2 cups) drinking coconut,
    almond or macadamia milk
90 g (3 oz/½ cup) quinoa, thoroughly rinsed
1 tablespoon chia seeds
2 teaspoons fresh ginger, finely chopped
1½ teaspoons ground cinnamon
½ teaspoon ground nutmeg
1 teaspoon natural vanilla extract
⅛ teaspoon ground cloves
stevia, to taste (optional)

Toppings
125 ml (4 fl oz/½ cup) tinned coconut milk
1 medium pear, thinly sliced
40 g (1½ oz/⅓ cup) walnuts, coarsely chopped
manuka honey, to serve (optional)

In a medium saucepan, combine the water and 375 ml (12½ fl oz/1½ cups) of the coconut milk and bring to the boil. Add the quinoa and reduce to a medium heat. Cook for 10–15 minutes until most of the liquid is absorbed and the quinoa's little 'tails' have sprouted. Add the remaining coconut milk, chia seeds, ginger, cinnamon, nutmeg, vanilla and cloves and stir to combine. Remove from the heat and stand for 5 minutes, or until the chia seeds have rehydrated and the porridge is creamy. Sweeten with stevia, if desired.

Serve topped with coconut milk, sliced pear and walnuts. Drizzle on some honey, if desired.

CARLA'S TIP To save time, you can mix the quinoa, chia seeds and spices and portion them into small containers for a quick, sugar-free breakfast reminiscent of instant oats. Just cook them with the water and coconut milk.

LOW-FODMAP OPTION Swap drinking coconut milk for almond or macadamia milk, and swap pear for 80 g (2¾ oz) blueberries. If you'd like some extra sweetness, use a little pure organic maple syrup instead of honey.

Breakfast

98   Gluten Free   Dairy Free   Vegetarian   Vegan Option   Stage 2 Friendly   Low-FODMAP Option

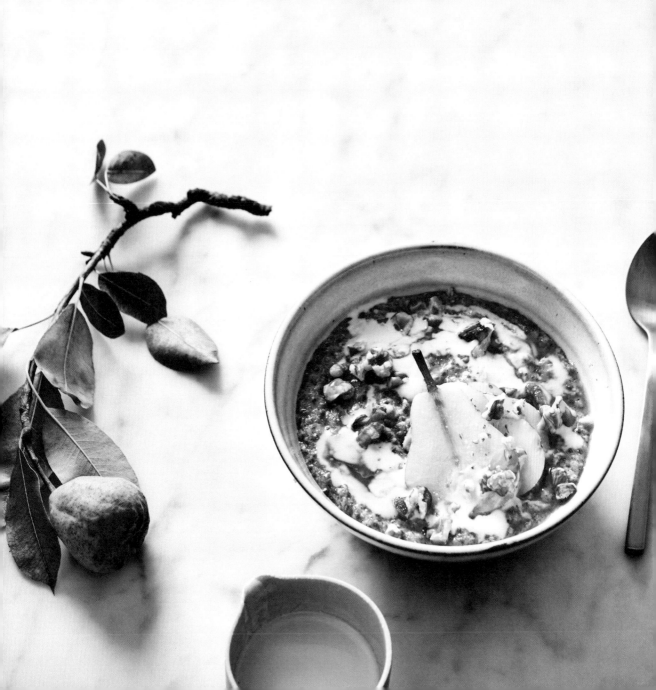

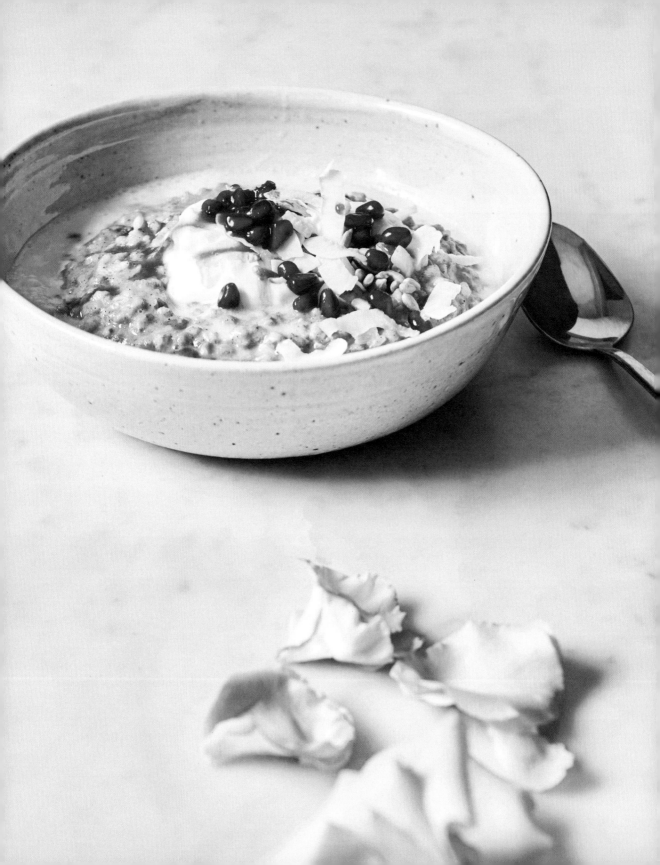

Sweet Potato, Miso & Buckwheat Porridge

This gutsy gluten-free porridge combines fibre- and protein-rich buckwheat with sweet potato to make a delicious, nourishing comfort food for you and your friendly microbes. Sweet potato contains insoluble fibre, helping to keep you regular, as well as pro-vitamin A, important for keeping your gut lining robust. Cinnamon and nutmeg bring a host of anti-inflammatory benefits, but the hero is in the topping. Pomegranate seeds have been shown to stimulate the growth of beneficial bacteria while inhibiting pathogenic bugs, helping to restore balance in the microbiota.

SERVES 4

150 g (5½ oz/¾ cup) buckwheat groats,
    washed & drained
splash of unpasteurised apple-cider vinegar
400 g (14 oz/1 medium) sweet potato, peeled & cut
    into 2 cm (¾ in) cubes
500 ml (17 fl oz/2 cups) drinking coconut,
    almond or macadamia milk
250 ml (8½ fl oz/1 cup) water
3 teaspoons white miso
1 teaspoon ground nutmeg
2 teaspoons ground cinnamon, plus extra for topping
1 teaspoon natural vanilla extract
stevia, equivalent to 2 teaspoons regular sugar,
    or to taste

Toppings
250 g (9 oz/1 cup) coconut yoghurt
35 g (1¼ oz/¼ cup) pomegranate seeds
30 g (1 oz/½ cup) coconut flakes
2 tablespoons sunflower kernels
manuka honey, for drizzling (optional)

Fill a small bowl up halfway with warm water. Add the buckwheat groats and vinegar and set aside in a warm place to soak for at least 2 (and up to 6) hours. Drain and rinse.

Steam the sweet potato for 10 minutes, or until tender, then mash into a purée (you can do this ahead of time and keep it in the refrigerator).

In a large saucepan, combine the coconut milk, water and buckwheat groats. Bring to the boil over a high heat, then reduce the heat and let simmer for 20 minutes, stirring occasionally, or until softened and tender.

Add the sweet potato, miso, nutmeg, cinnamon, vanilla extract and stevia. Stir continuously and cook for 3–4 more minutes. Add a little extra coconut milk or water to reach your desired porridge consistency.

Serve the porridge topped with coconut yoghurt, pomegranate seeds, coconut flakes and sunflower kernels, a sprinkling of cinnamon and a drizzle of manuka honey, as desired.

CARLA'S TIP Buckwheat porridge stores really well in the refrigerator. Divide any leftover porridge between jars and eat it cold or warm for a quick breakfast during the week. Cooling the sweet potato also increases its resistant starch, helping to produce short-chain fatty acids that help fight inflammation.

LOW-FODMAP OPTION Reduce the sweet potato to 300 g (10½ oz), swap the drinking coconut milk for unsweetened UHT coconut almond or macadamia milk, and swap the honey for some pure organic maple syrup.

Gluten Free   Dairy Free   Vegetarian   Vegan Option   Stage 2 Friendly   Low-FODMAP Option

Banana, Coconut & Turmeric Muffins

Muffins are a great on-the-go breakfast, but rather than eating the sugar-laden, store-bought version, why not make your own healthy ones? These muffins are satiating, and they're a good source of fibre and clean, sustainable energy. Bananas are a prebiotic food, assisting with the growth of beneficial bacteria, while pecans are full of fibre and rich in manganese, a mineral that helps activate digestive enzymes.

MAKES 12

4 free-range organic eggs, lightly beaten
300 g (10½ oz/about 2 medium) green (unripe)
    bananas, mashed
200 ml (7 fl oz) drinking coconut or nut-based milk
80 g (2¾ oz) unsalted butter, melted & cooled,
    or macadamia oil
1 teaspoon unpasteurised apple-cider vinegar
60 g (2 oz/½ cup) coconut flour
2 tablespoons buckwheat flour
1 teaspoon ground turmeric
1 teaspoon ground nutmeg
½ teaspoon freshly ground black pepper
1 teaspoon gluten-free baking powder
½ teaspoon bicarbonate of soda (baking soda)
stevia equal to 1 tablespoon of regular sugar
70 g (2½ oz/½ cup) pecans, roughly chopped
2 tablespoons cacao nibs, plus extra
    for garnish (optional)
250 g (9 oz/1 cup) coconut yoghurt,
    for garnish (optional)
20 g (¾ oz/⅓ cup) coconut flakes, lightly toasted,
    for garnish (optional)

Preheat the oven to 180°C (350°F/Gas Mark 4). Lightly grease and line a 12-hole standard muffin tin.

In a medium bowl, combine the eggs, bananas, coconut milk, butter or oil, and vinegar and stir well.

In a separate bowl, sift the coconut flour, buckwheat flour, turmeric, nutmeg, pepper, baking powder, bicarb soda and stevia and mix well. Add the dry ingredients to the egg mixture and mix well. Stir through the pecans and cacao nibs.

Spoon the batter into the prepared muffin tin, filling each one almost to the top, and bake for 20–25 minutes until golden brown, or until a skewer inserted into the centre comes out clean. Leave to cool in the tin for 10 minutes, then turn out onto a rack to cool completely.

Decorate each muffin with a dollop of coconut yoghurt, some toasted coconut and cacao nibs, if desired.

Undecorated muffins will keep in an airtight container in the refrigerator for up to 1 week, decorated ones for up to 3 days.

CARLA'S TIP Ripe bananas can also be used in these muffins; however, they will not contain as much digestive resistant starch, which is proven to be beneficial to your gut health.

Gluten Free   Dairy-Free Option   Vegetarian   Stage 4 Friendly

Herbed & Spiced Turmeric Eggs

Parsley and other herbs are very easy to grow. Having a herb garden, even if it is just on a window sill, exposes you to soil-based microbes and allows you to harvest your own fresh produce. This delightful, herbaceous, spicy breakfast offers a good dose of protein to set you up for the day and contains turmeric, an excellent gut healer, and cumin, great for increasing bile production to help digest fats. It's finished off with a sprinkling of sumac to give the eggs a piquant spark.

SERVES 2

6 free-range organic eggs
1 teaspoon ground turmeric
¼ teaspoon ground cumin
¼ teaspoon sea salt
¼ teaspoon freshly ground black pepper
1 tablespoon ghee or extra-virgin olive oil
1 large handful flat-leaf (Italian) parsley leaves,
   coarsely chopped
1 large handful coriander (cilantro) stems &
   leaves, coarsely chopped
50 g (1¾ oz) bitter lettuce, such as mizuna
   or rocket (arugula), to serve
1 tomato, sliced, to serve
½ long green chilli, finely sliced, to serve (optional)
1 teaspoon sumac, to serve

In a medium bowl, whisk the eggs, turmeric, cumin, salt and pepper until combined.

Melt the ghee in a medium non-stick frying pan over a low–medium heat. Add the egg mixture and cook, without stirring, for 30 seconds, or until the egg begins to set. Add the parsley and coriander and cook for another minute, stirring occasionally, until the egg starts to set in big curds but is still wet.

Serve immediately on beds of lettuce with tomato and sliced chilli, if desired, and sprinkle over a bit of sumac to serve.

CARLA'S TIP Scrambled eggs are so much creamier when you don't overcook them. Take them off the heat while they are still quite soft, as they will continue to cook. Think golden with a glistening surface, not pale with an omelette texture.

Gluten Free   Dairy-Free Option   Vegetarian   Stage 1 Friendly   Low FODMAP

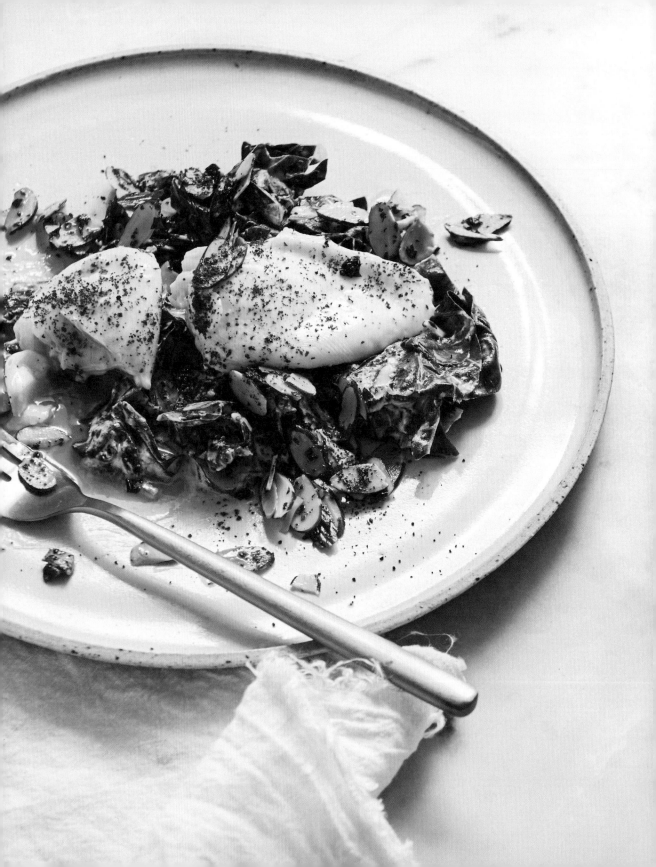

Sautéed Silverbeet, Sheep's Yoghurt & Poached Eggs

Green is always good. A recent study suggests that an enzyme found in dark-green leafy vegetables feeds beneficial gut bacteria while fending off pathogenic bacteria. Leafy greens also happen to be high in magnesium, which helps with bowel movements by relaxing the muscles of the intestinal wall. Eggs are a great source of B and D vitamins, zinc and selenium, all vital for healthy digestive function.

SERVES 2

splash of white vinegar
4 free-range organic eggs
60 ml (2 fl oz/¼ cup) ghee or extra-virgin olive oil
75 g (2¾ oz) silverbeet (Swiss chard), stems trimmed
    & leaves roughly chopped
180 g (6½ oz/¾ cup) sheep's yoghurt
1½ tablespoons freshly squeezed lemon juice
sea salt & freshly ground black pepper, to taste
2 tablespoons almond flakes
1 tablespoon oregano, finely chopped
1 teaspoon sumac, to serve

Bring a medium saucepan of water to a gentle simmer. Add a splash of vinegar.

Crack the eggs, one at a time, into a small bowl or ramekin, then gently slide them into the simmering vinegar water. Poach for 2–3 minutes until the whites are firm but the yolks are still soft. Remove them using a slotted spoon and set them on paper towel to drain.

Heat 1 tablespoon of the ghee in a large frying pan. Sauté the silverbeet leaves over a low heat until just wilted (refrigerate the stems for future recipes). Turn off the heat and add the yoghurt, lemon, salt and pepper to the pan, stirring to combine. Transfer the mixture to a bowl and cover to keep it warm.

Wipe out the pan with paper towel, then heat the remaining ghee over a medium–high heat. Add the almond flakes and oregano and toast them until crisp.

To serve, arrange the eggs on top of the silverbeet, then scatter over the toasted almonds and oregano and drizzle on any remaining ghee from the pan. Sprinkle with sumac.

CARLA'S TIP If you're missing your morning toast, try a slice of the fabulous gluten-free Prebiotic Superseed Bread (page 242).

Gluten Free   Vegetarian   Stage 4 Friendly

Stracciatella Savoury Breakfast Soup

I find having soup for breakfast the most nourishing way to start the day. I've swapped out cheese for nutritional yeast flakes in my version of this traditional Italian soup, making it dairy free and full of immune-boosting benefits. Both eggs and nutritional yeast contain B vitamins, which are vital for keeping the tissues of your digestive system healthy. Using chicken broth as a base ensures that your belly reaps the benefits of amino acid–rich collagen, important for maintaining a healthy gut lining. Add L-glutamine-rich eggs and you have a nutrient-dense breakfast with only four ingredients.

SERVES 4

1.5 litres (51 fl oz/6 cups) chicken Bone Broth or
    Vegetarian Broth (page 229), or store-bought stock
4 free-range organic eggs
3 large handfuls flat-leaf (Italian) parsley,
    roughly chopped
3 tablespoons nutritional yeast flakes
sea salt & freshly ground black pepper, to taste

Pour 60 ml (2 fl oz/¼ cup) of the broth into a medium bowl. Crack the eggs into the broth and whisk to combine. Stir in the parsley and nutritional yeast flakes.

Pour the remaining broth into a medium saucepan and bring to the boil, then reduce to a gentle simmer. Whisking continuously, slowly pour in the egg mixture. The egg will form small curds as it cooks. Season with salt and pepper to serve.

CARLA'S TIP Add some silverbeet (Swiss chard), kale or spinach for an extra hit of antioxidants and fibre. Lemon juice is also a zesty, healthful addition.

Gluten Free   Dairy Free   Vegetarian Option   Stage 1 Friendly   Low FODMAP

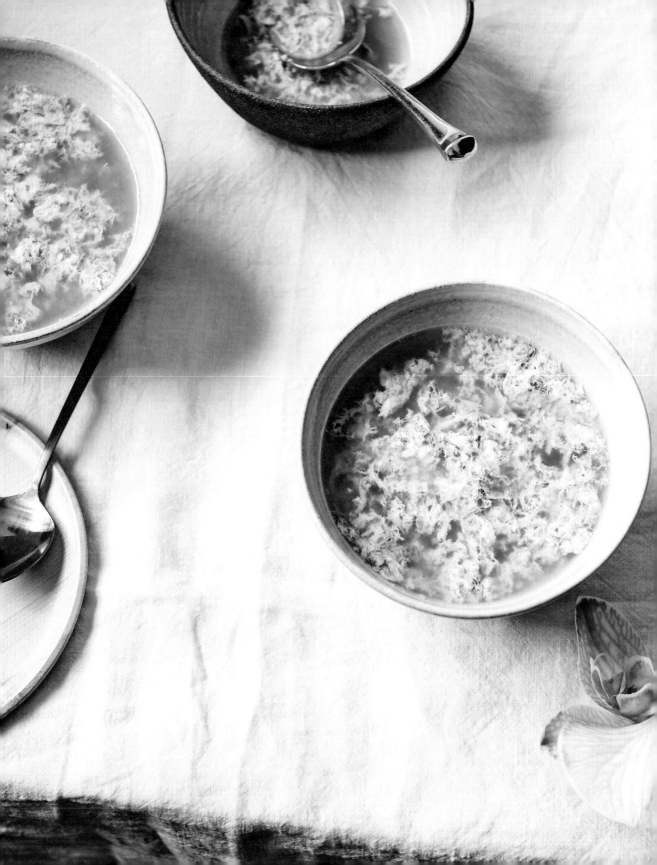

Kimchi, Avocado & Spinach Omelette

This quick breakfast boasts one of my favourite fermented foods: kimchi. With loads of spice and flavour and packed with cruciferous vegetables, garlic and ginger, kimchi acts as a potent pre-, pro- and postbiotic in the gut. More and more research supports its ability to promote healthy digestion, immune function and skin health.

SERVES 2 (Makes 2 omelettes)

6 free-range organic eggs
3 teaspoons ghee or extra-virgin olive oil
4 large handfuls baby spinach
100 g (3½ oz/½ cup) kimchi, sliced
1 ripe avocado, stone removed, sliced

Using a fork, lightly beat the eggs in a medium bowl until the whites start marbling through the yolks.

Preheat a large frying pan over a medium–high heat. To make the first omelette, add 1 teaspoon of the ghee to the hot pan and swirl to coat it. Pour half of the egg mixture into the pan, tilting it to coat the base and form a thin omelette. Cook for 20–30 seconds until golden and just set. Slide the omelette onto a large serving plate and cover to keep warm. Repeat the process with the remaining egg mixture and 1 teaspoon of ghee.

To prepare the filling, melt the remaining teaspoon of ghee in the pan over a medium heat. Add the spinach and toss until it wilts. Remove the pan from the heat, add the kimchi, and toss to combine.

To assemble, arrange slices of avocado on top of each omelette and top with spinach and kimchi filling. Serve immediately.

CARLA'S TIP This omelette is delicious when paired with Low-FODMAP Charcoal Flatbread (page 235), Turmeric Roti (page 234) or Prebiotic Superseed Bread (page 242).

LOW-FODMAP OPTION Swap kimchi and avocado for no more than 65 g (2¼ oz) zucchini (courgette) per serve. You can also add some grated carrot, sliced red capsicum (bell pepper), bean sprouts or the green part of spring onion (scallion).

Gluten Free   Dairy-Free Option   Vegetarian   Stage 3 Friendly   Low-FODMAP Option

Romesco Baked Eggs

I often make a big batch of romesco and divvy it up into small containers to freeze. It makes baked eggs so easy: just heat up the sauce, crack in a couple of eggs, sprinkle over some herbs and bake. This recipe makes breakfast in the healing stage interesting and delicious. Capsicum (bell pepper), the star in this Spanish favourite, works well alongside carrots. They're rich in anti-inflammatory flavonoids: plant compounds that studies show may help promote microbial diversity.

SERVES 2

1 teaspoon extra-virgin olive oil, plus extra
    for brushing & drizzling
375 ml (12½ fl oz/1½ cups) Nut-Free
    Roasted Romesco (page 241)
125 ml (4½ fl oz/½ cup) water
150 g (5½ oz) baby spinach
4 free-range organic eggs
freshly chopped basil or parsley, for sprinkling
freshly ground black pepper, to serve

Preheat the oven to 200°C (400°F/Gas Mark 6). Brush two 3.5 cm (1½ in) deep, 500 ml (17 fl oz/ 2 cups) capacity ovenproof dishes with olive oil. Alternatively you can use two small (14 cm/5½ in) ovenproof frying pans.

Pour the romesco and water into a medium saucepan and bring to a simmer over a low–medium heat.

Meanwhile, heat the oil in a medium frying pan over a low–medium heat. Add the spinach and cook until just wilted.

Divide the sauce between the prepared dishes. Arrange the spinach on top. Make two hollows in the sauce in each dish, then crack the eggs into the hollows.

Bake for 8–10 minutes until the whites are set but the yolks are still runny, or until cooked to your liking.

Serve the eggs drizzled with olive oil and topped with herbs and freshly ground black pepper.

CARLA'S TIP Capsicum (bell pepper) contains capsaicin, which can trigger symptoms in some individuals with irritable bowel syndrome. If you notice your symptoms start to flare up, limit intake.

Gluten Free   Dairy Free   Vegetarian   Stage 1 Friendly   Low FODMAP

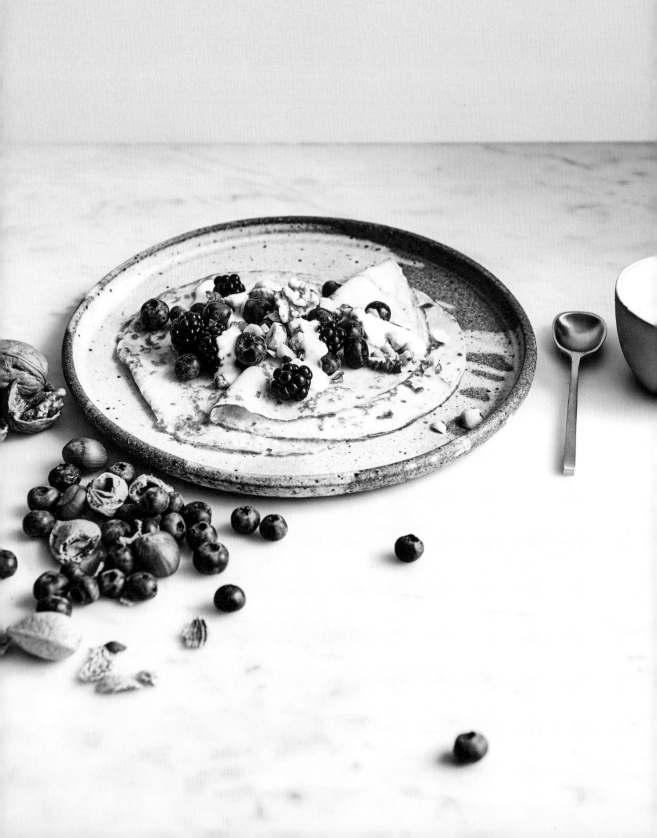

Coconut Crêpes
with Coconut Yoghurt & Berries

Crêpes are always a good idea, especially when they're packed full of coconutey goodness. In our house, these are a Sunday morning favourite. Apart from being rich in healthy fats, coconut milk and/or yoghurt are great dairy-free alternatives for those who struggle to digest whole-milk dairy. Blackberries and blueberries are both low-GI fruits, and are anti-inflammatory and antioxidant rich.

SERVES 4 (Makes 12 x 20 cm/8 in crêpes)

60 g (2 oz/½ cup) coconut flour
60 g (2 oz/½ cup) arrowroot
6 free-range organic eggs
375 ml (12½ fl oz/1½ cups) almond milk
ghee or extra-virgin coconut oil, for greasing

Toppings
500 g (1 lb 2 oz/2 cups) coconut yoghurt
250 g (9 oz) blueberries
250 g (9 oz) blackberries
75 g (2¾ oz/½ cup) pomegranate seeds (optional)
70 g (2½ oz/½ cup) coarsely chopped mixed nuts,
     such as pecans, hazelnuts, walnuts & almonds

To prepare the crêpes, whisk the coconut flour and arrowroot in a medium bowl. In a separate bowl, whisk the eggs and almond milk until well combined. Gradually pour the wet into the dry ingredients, whisking continuously to form a smooth batter. Cover and refrigerate for 30 minutes to allow the coconut flour to rehydrate.

Heat a 20 cm (8 in) non-stick saucepan over a medium heat. Dip a paper towel into ghee or coconut oil and rub it over the hot pan to lightly grease it. Pour 60 ml (2 fl oz/¼ cup) batter into the pan and swirl to coat in an even layer. Cook the crêpe for 30–60 seconds until the surface dries out and the underside is lacy and golden. Flip and cook for another 20 seconds, or until golden. Transfer to a plate, cover to keep warm and set aside. Repeat the process with the remaining batter.

Serve the crêpes topped with coconut yoghurt, berries, nuts and pomegranate seeds, if desired. The crêpes can be made in advance and stored in the refrigerator for up to 1 week or frozen for up to 3 months.

CARLA'S TIP   Enjoy these crêpes with a healthy, polyphenol-rich chocolate sauce made with cacao: just combine 20 g (¾ oz) raw cacao powder, 2 teaspoons coconut oil, 2 dates (pitted and coarsely chopped), 1 tablespoon pure organic maple syrup, 125 ml (4 fl oz/½ cup) boiling water and a pinch of sea salt, and blend.

Gluten Free   Vegetarian   Dairy-Free Option   Stage 3 Friendly

Sri Lankan Scrambled Eggs with Coconut Sambol

Pol Sambol is a wonderfully flavoursome Sri Lankan dish prepared with grated coconut and used as an accompaniment to meals. While coconut has a host of health benefits on its own, it gets an extra boost of healthy goodness here with anti-inflammatory ginger, garlic and mustard seeds, all beneficial for supporting digestive health and detoxing your system.

SERVES 2

Coconut Sambol
80 g (2¾ oz/1 cup) shredded coconut
2 teaspoons ghee or extra-virgin olive oil
1 shallot, finely sliced
3 teaspoons fresh ginger, finely chopped
1 garlic clove, finely chopped
½ green chilli, thinly sliced
6 curry leaves, dried or fresh
¼ teaspoon mustard seeds
1½ tablespoons freshly squeezed lime juice
sea salt & freshly ground black pepper, to taste

Sri Lankan Scrambled Eggs
2 tablespoons ghee or extra-virgin olive oil
4 free-range organic eggs, lightly beaten
2 large handfuls coriander (cilantro),
    stems & leaves, to serve
2 Turmeric Roti (page 234), warmed, to serve

To prepare the coconut sambol, soak the coconut in a bowl of cold water for 10 minutes, then drain and set aside.

Heat the ghee in a medium frying pan over a medium heat. Add the shallot, ginger and garlic and sauté for 1 minute, or until softened. Add the chilli, curry leaves and mustard seeds and cook, stirring occasionally, until the seeds begin to pop. Add the coconut and stir to combine. Cook for 2 minutes, or until heated through. Add the lime juice, salt and pepper and stir to combine. Cover the dish to keep warm and set aside.

To make the Sri Lankan scrambled eggs, melt the ghee in a small non-stick saucepan over a low–medium heat. Let the eggs cook for 30 seconds without stirring, or until they begin to set. Cook for another minute, stirring occasionally, until the egg sets in big curds but is still moist. Add the coconut sambol and the coriander and gently stir through.

Serve with Turmeric Roti.

CARLA'S TIP You can also swap the turmeric roti for Prebiotic Superseed Bread (page 242).

LOW-FODMAP OPTION Reduce the shredded coconut to 60 g (2 oz/¾ cup). Omit the shallot and garlic and use the green part of two spring onions (scallions) instead.

Gluten Free   Dairy-Free Option   Vegetarian   Stage 4 Friendly   Low-FODMAP Option

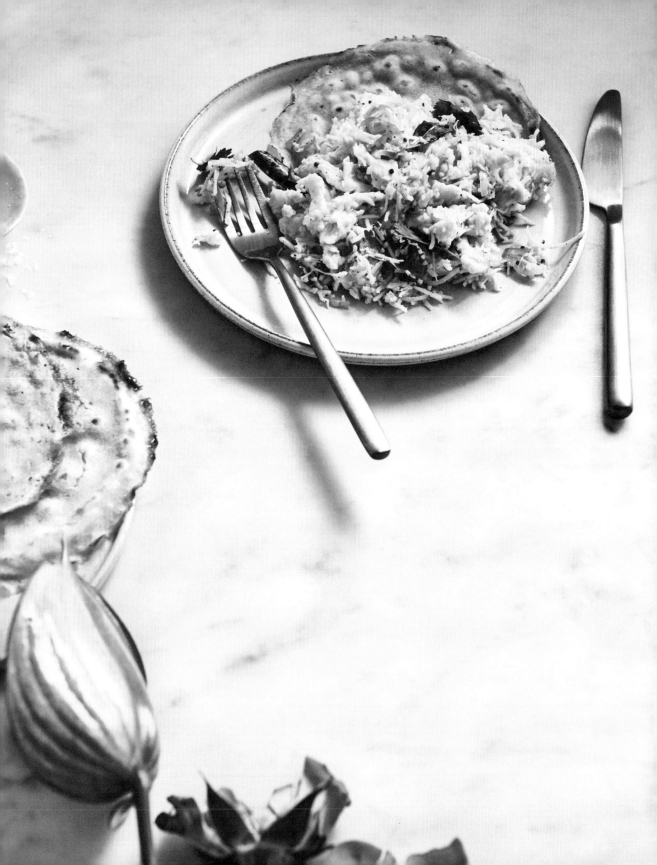

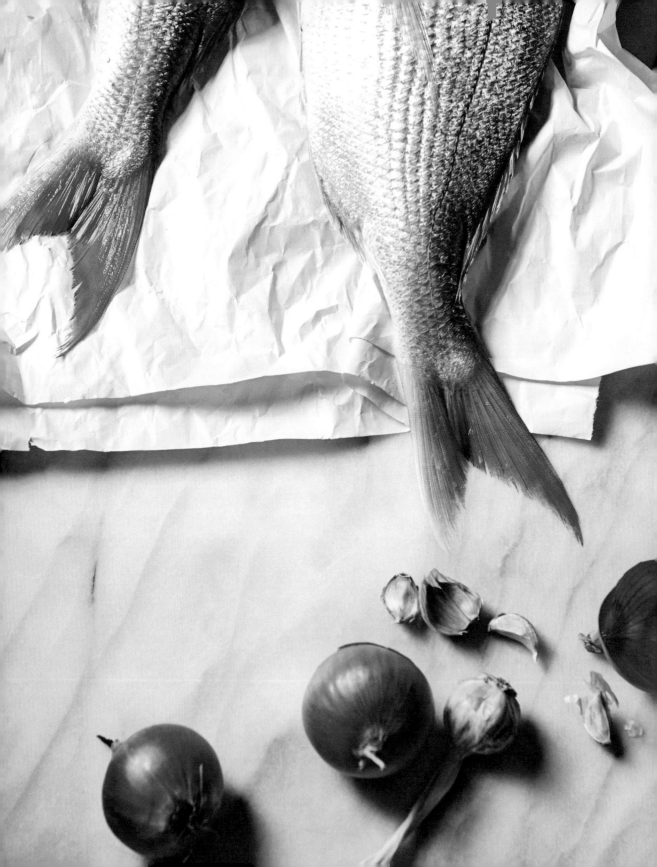

Lunch & Dinner

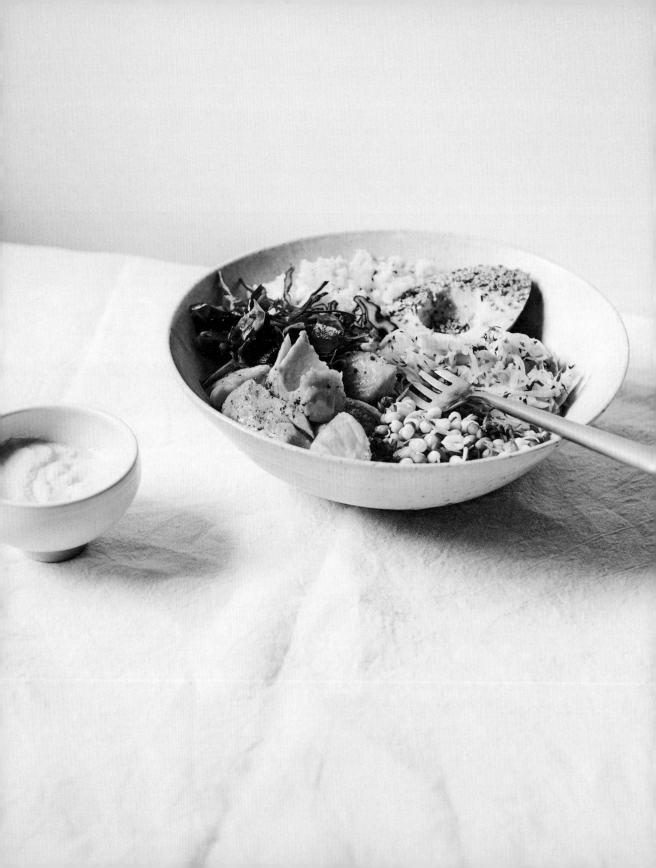

Salmon Lunch Bowl

Lunch bowls make organising your midday meal effortless, and they are a brilliant way to ensure you are getting a balanced meal with lots of vegetables, a few complex carbs, good fats and some protein. This recipe is rich in omega-3s, protein and fermented goodness. Homemade Sauerkraut (page 236), or the store-bought unpasteurised version, contains a host of beneficial pro-, pre- and postbiotics. Salmon, eggs and red cabbage are all great sources of L-glutamine, an amino acid that helps strengthen the gut lining and prevent leaky gut syndrome.

SERVES 2

2 tablespoons dried instant wakame flakes
½ quantity Cauliflower Rice (page 240)
1 handful mint, coarsely chopped
1 handful dill, coarsely chopped
80 g (2¾ oz/1 cup) finely shredded red cabbage
1 handful mung bean sprouts
2 × 210 g (7½ oz) tins Alaskan red salmon or sardines
2 soft-boiled eggs, halved
1 medium ripe avocado, halved & flesh scooped out
100 g (3½ oz/½ cup) Sauerkraut with Carrot,
    Caraway Seeds & Juniper Berries (page 236)
80 ml (2½ fl oz/⅓ cup) Miso, Tahini & Umeboshi
    Dressing (page 245)

Soak the wakame in cold water for 10 minutes, or until rehydrated. Drain and set aside.

In a medium bowl, combine the cauliflower rice, mint and dill.

Divide the cauliflower rice, cabbage and mung bean sprouts between two serving bowls. Top with salmon, soft-boiled eggs, avocado, wakame and sauerkraut. Drizzle with Miso, Tahini & Umeboshi Dressing to serve.

CARLA'S TIP If you are in Stage 4 of the Gut Guide, add a sprinkling of Coriander, Chilli & Fennel Salt (page 239) – it's great for digestion and adds depth of flavour. Sliced steamed chicken or leftover baked or steamed fish can be substituted for the tinned fish.

Baked Yoghurt & Herb Salmon
with Fennel & Lemon

It's no secret that salmon is rich in omega-3 fatty acids, which offer a range of health-related benefits. What scientists have recently discovered, though, is that these benefits may be due in part to increases in butyrate-producing bacteria. Butyrate plays a key role in maintaining optimal gut health. What better reason to add this recipe to your weekly repertoire, paired here with fennel, lemon and mint to help aid digestion.

SERVES 4

extra-virgin olive oil, for drizzling
190 g (6½ oz, 1 small) fennel bulb, halved, trimmed,
    cored & thinly sliced
1 leek, green part only
2 large handfuls dill, coarsely chopped,
    plus extra to serve
60 ml (2 fl oz/¼ cup) freshly squeezed lemon juice
    & finely grated zest of 1 unwaxed lemon
sea salt & freshly ground black pepper, to taste
4 × 150–200 g (5½–7 oz) skinless centre-cut salmon
    fillets, pin-boned
125 g (4½ oz/½ cup) goat's or sheep's yoghurt
1 large handful mint, coarsely chopped,
    plus extra to serve
35 g (1¼ oz/¼ cup) pine nuts, lightly toasted

Preheat the oven to 200°C (400°F/Gas Mark 6).

Drizzle some olive oil into the bottom of a 30 cm × 20 cm (12 in × 8 in) baking dish. Add the fennel, leek and half of the dill. Drizzle with a little more oil and half the lemon juice. Season with salt and pepper. Toss to combine. Cook in the oven for 10 minutes, or until the vegetables begin to soften.

Remove the dish from the oven and arrange the salmon pieces on top of the vegetables. Drizzle with some oil, pour over a little more lemon juice and season with salt and pepper. Top each salmon fillet with a dollop of yoghurt, spreading it over the surface in an even layer. Scatter with mint, some dill and the lemon zest. Return the dish to the oven and bake for another 10 minutes, or until the salmon is almost completely cooked through (or until cooked to your liking).

Serve the fish scattered with more mint, the remaining dill, pine nuts and a drizzle of extra-virgin olive oil.

CARLA'S TIP This dish pairs perfectly with roasted cherry tomatoes. Ensure you keep them under 75 g (2¾ oz) per serve if you are wanting a low-FODMAP meal.

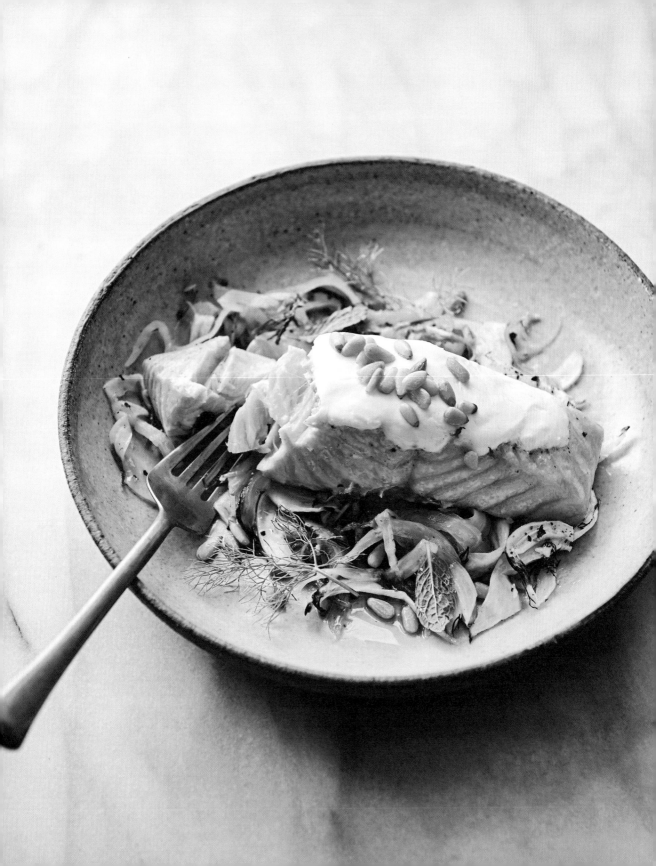

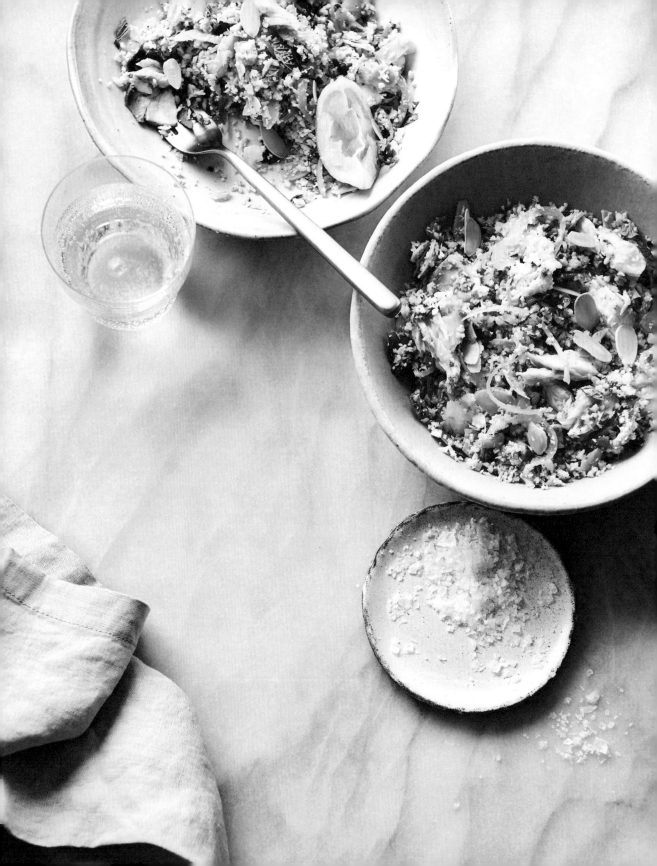

Spiced Barramundi & Masala Fried 'Rice'

I've always had a soft spot for garam masala, both for its spicy-but-sweet undertones and for how easy it is to add to fish, chicken, a stew or rice. When I feel like something a little lighter for dinner, I find some cauliflower 'rice' is the perfect happy medium for being both satiating and easy on my digestion. Cauliflower is high in anti-inflammatory vitamin C and rich in glucosinolates, which stimulate our body's natural antioxidant system. I love to add an egg fried in a little ghee or coconut oil on top with a smattering of chilli sauce.

SERVES 2

60 ml (2 fl oz/¼ cup) ghee, melted,
    or extra-virgin olive oil
2 teaspoons freshly squeezed lemon juice
1 teaspoon garam masala
⅛ teaspoon ground turmeric
⅛ teaspoon chilli powder
⅛ teaspoon freshly ground black pepper
300 g (10½ oz) skinless barramundi fillet
lemon wedges, to serve

Masala Fried 'Rice'

400 g (14 oz) cauliflower, cut into small florets
2 tablespoons ghee or extra-virgin olive oil
1 medium onion, thinly sliced
20 g (¾ oz/¼ cup) flaked almonds
2 teaspoons fresh ginger, finely chopped
2 garlic cloves, finely chopped
1 long green chilli, seeded & finely sliced
½ teaspoon garam masala
⅛ teaspoon ground turmeric
⅛ teaspoon chilli powder
1 handful coriander (cilantro) stems & leaves,
    coarsely chopped
1 handful mint, coarsely chopped
1 handful flat-leaf (Italian) parsley leaves,
    coarsely chopped
sea salt & freshly ground black pepper, to taste

Recipe continues >

Gluten Free   Dairy-Free Option   Stage 4 Friendly   Low-FODMAP Option

Preheat the oven to 200°C (400°F/Gas Mark 6) and line a baking tray with baking paper.

Combine the ghee, lemon juice and spices in a medium bowl. Add the barramundi and rub the spice mixture over the fish to coat. Cover and refrigerate for 15 minutes.

Place the fish on the pre-lined tray. Bake in the oven for 15–20 minutes until it is just cooked through and flakes easily. Remove from the oven, cover to keep warm and set aside.

While the fish is cooking, prepare the fried 'rice'. Blend the cauliflower in a food processor until it forms rice-sized grains.

Heat 1 tablespoon of the ghee in a large frying pan over a high–medium heat. Add the onion and cook until it caramelises to a dark brown colour, but isn't burnt. Transfer to a bowl and set aside.

Heat the remaining ghee in the pan and cook the almonds for 1–2 minutes until they begin to turn golden. Add the ginger, garlic, chilli, garam masala, turmeric and chilli powder and cook for 1 minute, or until the almonds are golden, the ginger and garlic have softened and the spices are fragrant. Add the mix to the bowl with the onions.

Add the cauliflower rice to the pan and cook on a medium–high heat, stirring frequently, for 3–4 minutes until the cauliflower is just tender and heated through. Stir through the onion, almond and spice mix to combine.

Flake the fish into bite-sized chunks and add it to the cauliflower rice along with the coriander, mint and parsley. Stir to combine. Season with salt and pepper and serve with some lemon wedges.

CARLA'S TIP Garam masala is an Indian spice mix traditionally containing pepper, cloves, cinnamon, nutmeg, cardamom, bay leaf, cumin and coriander. If you have these spices on hand at home, get the pestle and mortar out and have a go at making your own.

LOW-FODMAP OPTION Swap the Masala Fried Rice for Gut-Healing Turmeric & Parsley Tabouleh (page 198). From Stage 2 onwards, cauliflower 'rice' can be substituted for 285 g (10 oz/1½ cups) cooked white basmati rice. Replace the onion with the green part of 3 spring onions (scallions), thinly sliced. Omit the garlic.

Grilled Sardines on Fried Buckwheat Cakes with Silverbeet & Harissa

Sardines may not be everyone's cup of tea, but I'm hoping this delicious recipe will change your mind. With research showing that omega-3 fats are highly beneficial for gut health, sardines are a great way to incorporate these healthy fats without the health-compromising levels of mercury found in other types of fish and seafood. They're also rich in selenium, a mineral that helps heal the gut and is needed for our body's production of the powerful antioxidant glutathione.

SERVES 4

12–16 medium fresh sardine fillets, butterflied
coconut or extra-virgin olive oil, for drizzling
sea salt & freshly ground black pepper, to taste
1½ tablespoons ghee or extra-virgin olive oil
150 g (5½ oz) silverbeet (Swiss chard), shredded
1½ tablespoons freshly squeezed lemon juice

Harissa (Makes 250 ml/8½ fl oz/1 cup)
1 red capsicum (bell pepper)
60 g (2 oz, about 3) long red chillies
2 garlic cloves, peeled
½ teaspoon sea salt
½ teaspoon ground cumin
½ teaspoon ground coriander
¼ teaspoon ground caraway seeds
2 tablespoons extra-virgin olive oil,
    plus extra for storage
2 teaspoons unpasteurised apple-cider vinegar

Fried Buckwheat Cakes
150 g (5½ oz/¾ cup) buckwheat groats
splash of unpasteurised apple-cider vinegar
560 ml (19 fl oz/2¼ cups) chicken Bone Broth or
    Vegetarian Broth (page 229), or store-bought stock
2½ tablespoons nutritional yeast flakes
sea salt & freshly ground black pepper, to taste
30 g (1 oz/¼ cup) arrowroot, for coating
1 large free-range organic egg, lightly beaten with
    a splash of nut-based milk
100 g (3½ oz/1 cup) quinoa flakes
coconut oil, for shallow frying

CARLA'S TIP If you don't have time to make fried buckwheat cakes, put the sardines and sauce on some Low-FODMAP Charcoal Flatbread (page 235) – think sardines on toast.

LOW-FODMAP OPTION To make this recipe low FODMAP, omit the garlic.

Recipe continues >

Gluten Free   Dairy-Free Option   Stage 2 Friendly   Low-FODMAP Option

Preheat the oven to 200°C (400°F/Gas Mark 6). Line a baking tray with baking paper.

To prepare the buckwheat groats, fill a small bowl up halfway with warm water. Add the buckwheat groats and vinegar and set aside in a warm place to soak for at least 2 (and up to 6) hours. Drain and rinse.

To make the harissa sauce, place the capsicum on the lined baking tray and roast for 30 minutes. Add the chillies to the tray and roast for a further 15–20 minutes until the skins are blistered and everything has softened and begun to lose shape. Transfer the capsicum and chillies to a bowl, cover and set aside to cool. Once cooled, peel and de-seed. Blend with the remaining ingredients in a food processor until smooth. Transfer the sauce to a bowl, cover and set aside.

To make the buckwheat cakes, lightly grease and line a 20 cm (8 in) square cake tin with baking paper. Put the buckwheat in a small saucepan with the chicken broth and bring to the boil. Reduce to a simmer and cook, stirring occasionally, for 25–30 minutes, or until the buckwheat is tender and has turned into a creamy porridge consistency. Add the yeast, salt and pepper and stir to combine.

Transfer half of the buckwheat mixture to a food processor and blend until smooth. Return it to the saucepan and stir through the remaining buckwheat mixture. Pour the mix into the prepared tin and spread out to form a smooth, even surface. Cover with plastic wrap and refrigerate for 20 minutes, or until firmly set. Turn it out onto a clean chopping board, then cut into 12 even-sized pieces.

Put the arrowroot, egg wash and quinoa flakes into separate bowls in preparation for crumbing the buckwheat. Coat each piece with some arrowroot, shaking off any excess, then dip into the egg wash. Lastly, coat with quinoa flakes and press firmly to secure.

Pour coconut oil into a medium frying pan to a depth of 2 cm (¾ in). Place over a medium heat and heat until a quinoa flake dropped in floats straight to the surface. Fry the buckwheat cakes for 2–3 minutes on each side until golden brown. Transfer to paper towel to drain, then cover to keep warm.

To make the sardines, heat a large frying pan over a medium–high heat. Drizzle the sardines with oil and season with salt and pepper. Grill for 2 minutes on each side, or until golden brown and just cooked through. Transfer to a plate and cover to keep warm.

Reduce the temperature to a low–medium heat. Wipe the pan using paper towel. Melt the ghee and add the silverbeet. Cook until just wilted. Pour in the lemon juice and toss to coat. Season with salt and pepper.

Serve the sardines with a fried buckwheat cake, some sautéed silverbeet and topped with harissa sauce.

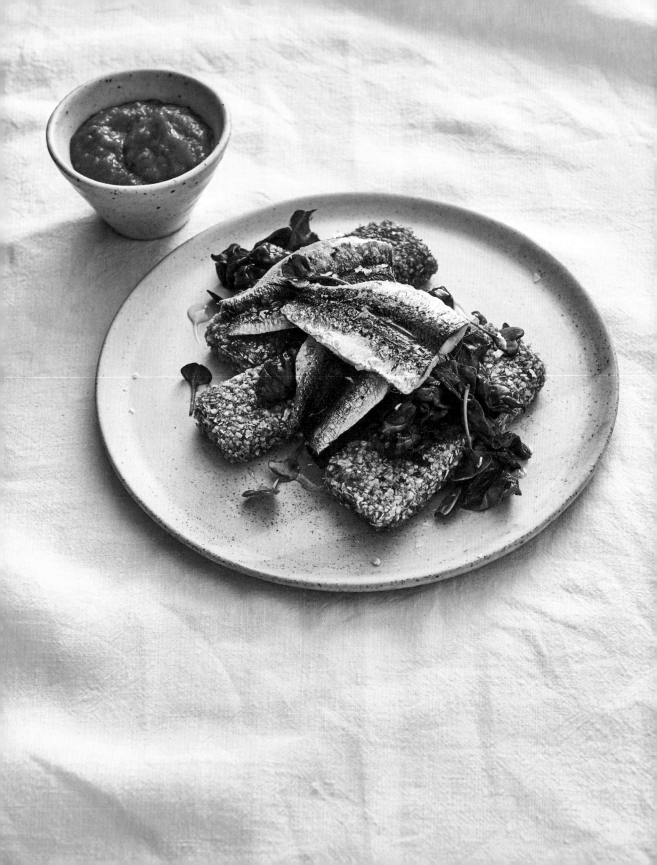

Tamarind Fish Curry

Curries are rich in all of those lovely aromatic and anti-inflammatory spices such as cumin, fennel, turmeric and cayenne. But if you want to take your curry to the next level, the sweet-and-sour flavours of tamarind purée are distinctive and delicious. Historically used to treat stomach problems, tamarind contains both soluble and insoluble fibre, maintaining digestive regularity and feeding the beneficial bacteria in your gut. The tartness of the pulp is balanced beautifully with the sweet flesh of the barramundi and the earthiness of the spices.

SERVES 2

2 tablespoons ghee or extra-virgin olive oil
1 medium onion, thinly sliced
1½ tablespoons fresh ginger, finely chopped
1 garlic clove, peeled
8 curry leaves, dried or fresh
½ teaspoon yellow mustard seeds
2 medium tomatoes, diced
2 tablespoons seedless tamarind purée
250 ml (8½ fl oz/1 cup) water
sea salt, to taste
300 g (10½ oz) skinless barramundi fillet,
    cut into large (about 8 cm/3¼ in) chunks
1 large handful coriander (cilantro) stems & leaves,
    coarsely chopped, to serve
Cauliflower Rice (page 240), to serve
Turmeric Roti (page 234), to serve (optional)

Curry Paste
2 tablespoons shredded coconut
1 teaspoon coriander seeds
½ teaspoon cumin seeds
½ teaspoon fennel seeds
1½ tablespoons ghee or extra-virgin olive oil
¼ teaspoon ground cinnamon
¼ teaspoon ground turmeric
⅛ teaspoon cayenne pepper

To prepare the curry paste, toast the coconut and coriander, cumin and fennel seeds in a small pan over a low–medium heat for 1 minute, or until golden. Grind with a spice grinder or mortar and pestle, then transfer to a small bowl. Add the ghee and remaining spices and blend to form a paste. Set aside.

Heat the ghee in a large frying pan over a low–medium heat. Cook the onion, ginger and garlic for 2–3 minutes until softened. Add the curry paste, curry leaves and mustard seeds and cook for about 30 seconds, or until the dish is fragrant and the mustard seeds begin to pop. Add the tomato and tamarind and stir to combine. Gradually pour in the water and bring to the boil. Reduce the curry to a simmer and cook for 15–20 minutes, or until reduced by half. Season with some salt.

Add the barramundi, cover and gently simmer for 6–7 minutes, or until just cooked through. Shake the pan occasionally to ensure the fish cooks evenly.

Scatter with coriander and serve with some Cauliflower Rice and Turmeric Roti, if desired.

CARLA'S TIP For a vegetarian version, swap the fish for 100 g (3½ oz/½ cup) mung beans or yellow split peas. Add them with the tomato and tamarind plus an extra 250 ml (8½ fl oz/1 cup) water and simmer for 30 minutes, or until the beans/peas are cooked through, but still a little tender.

Gluten Free   Dairy-Free Option   Vegetarian Option   Vegan Option   Stage 2 Friendly

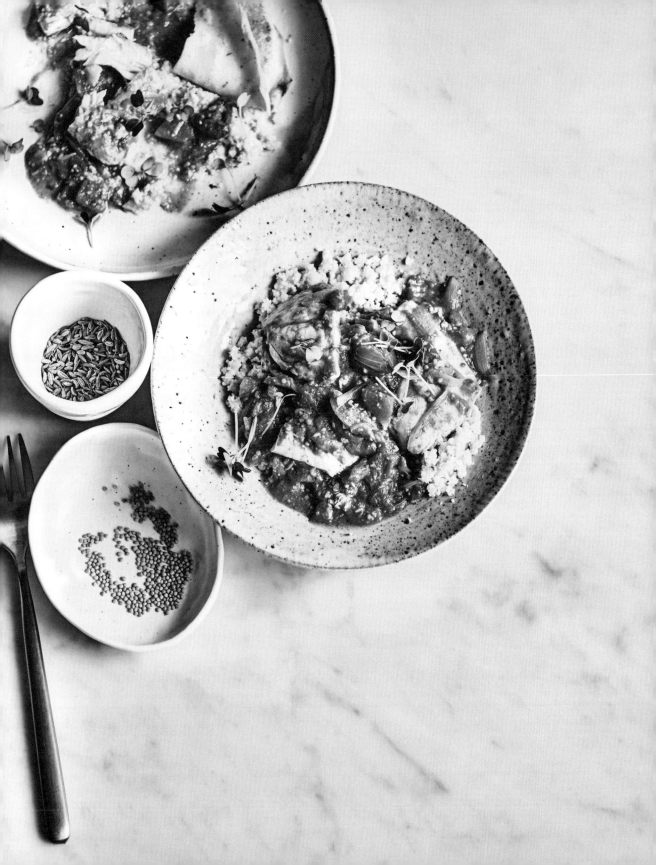

Kingfish Ceviche, Spiced Coconut & Tamarind Egg Bowl

When it comes to sharing nutrients with your microbiome, this is the perfect meal. Swapping sashimi for ceviche is a great way to enjoy 'raw' fish without the risk of harmful bacteria. The curing process, which uses lime and/or lemon juice, 'cooks' the ceviche and acts as a digestive aid, stimulating the initial stages of protein breakdown. The spiced coconut and tamarind eggs take the lunch bowl concept to new culinary heights with their delicious mix of spicy, sweet and sour, and crunchy.

SERVES 4

135 g (5 oz/¾ cup) quinoa, thoroughly rinsed
375 ml (12½ fl oz/1½ cups) water
8 g (¼ oz/⅓ cup) dried instant wakame flakes
400 g (14 oz) sashimi-grade kingfish
1½ tablespoons freshly squeezed lime juice
60 ml (2 fl oz/¼ cup) freshly squeezed lemon juice
2 tablespoons extra-virgin olive oil
sea salt & freshly ground black pepper, to taste
400 g (14 oz, about 1 bunch) kale, stems removed, leaves coarsely chopped
150 g (5½ oz/1 cup) Sauerkraut with Carrot, Caraway Seeds & Juniper Berries (low-FODMAP option, page 236)
tamari, to serve

Spiced Coconut & Tamarind Eggs
4 free-range organic eggs
60 g (2 oz/¾ cup) shredded coconut, lightly toasted
2 teaspoons coriander seeds, toasted & coarsely ground
2 teaspoons fennel seeds, toasted & coarsely ground
1 teaspoon chilli flakes
¼ teaspoon sea salt
2 tablespoons seedless tamarind purée

CARLA'S TIP If you're not partial to quinoa, swap it for 285 g (10 oz/1½ cups) cooked white basmati rice instead.

In a medium saucepan, combine the quinoa and water and bring to the boil. Cover and reduce to a gentle simmer for 15 minutes, cooking the quinoa until almost all of the water has been absorbed. Remove from the heat, then let sit, covered, for another 5 minutes, or until the quinoa's 'tails' have sprouted and the remaining water has been absorbed.

Soak the wakame in cold water for 5 minutes, or until rehydrated. Drain and set aside.

To make the eggs, cover with cold water in a small saucepan. Bring the water to a simmer over a low–medium heat. Cook the eggs for 3 minutes, then submerge in ice water. Once cooled slightly, peel.

In a bowl, toss the toasted coconut, coriander seeds, fennel seeds, chilli flakes and salt. Brush the eggs with tamarind purée, then roll in the spiced coconut mixture. Set aside.

Using a sharp knife, thinly slice the kingfish across the grain. Combine in a bowl with the lime juice, half the lemon juice, 1 tablespoon of the oil and some salt and black pepper. Cover and allow to marinate for 2–3 minutes.

Heat the remaining oil in a medium frying pan over a medium–high heat. Add the kale and the rest of the lemon juice and cook, stirring occasionally, for 2–3 minutes, or until wilted.

To assemble, divide the quinoa between serving bowls and arrange the kingfish ceviche, kale, wakame, sauerkraut and eggs on top. Drizzle with some tamari to serve.

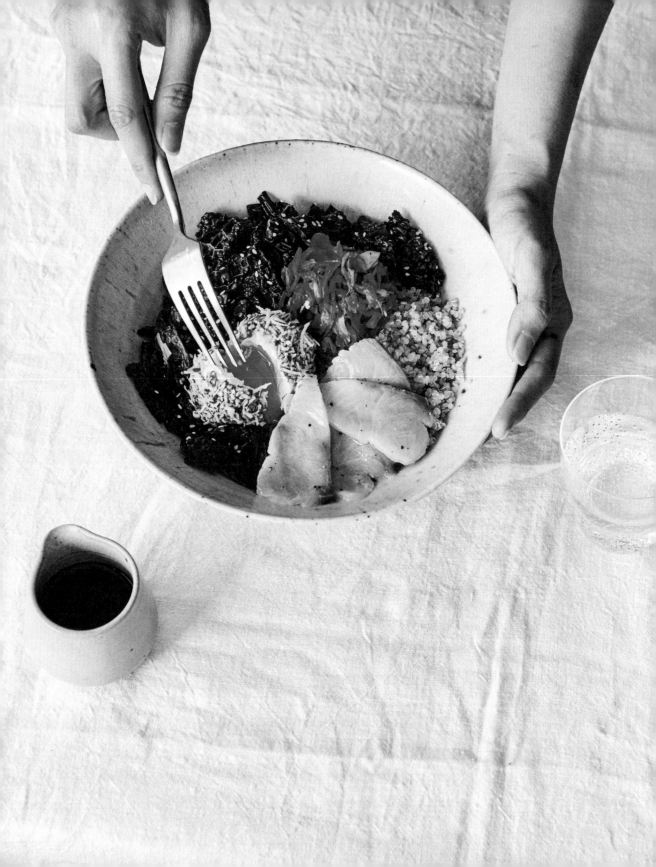

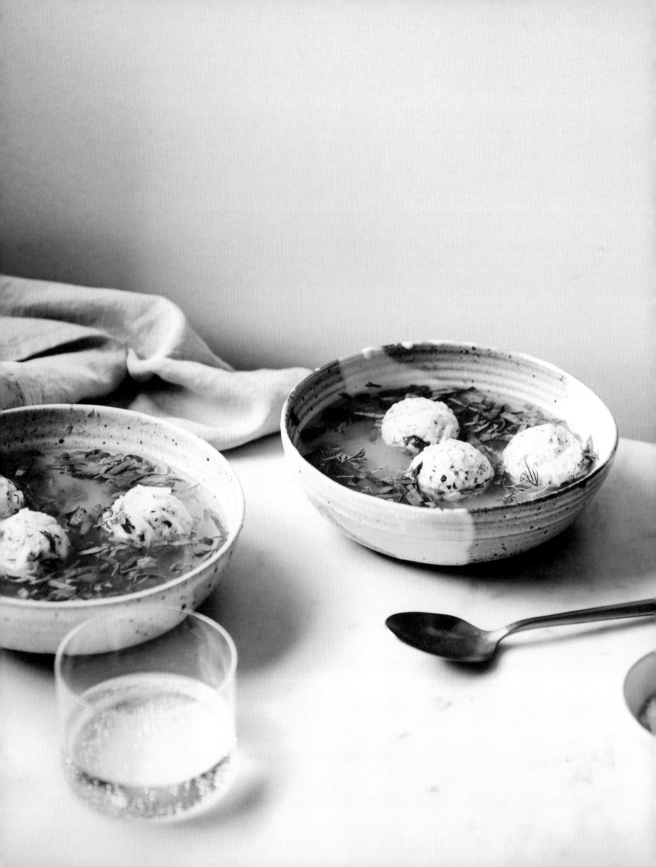

Dill-Infused Fish, Leek & Spinach Soup

I love this soup and eat it regularly. It's flavoursome, cleansing, and gentle on your digestive system. With bitter greens such as spinach to stimulate digestion, and generous clippings of anti-inflammatory herbs such as dill and parsley, used in both the broth and the patties, this soup is perfect for the Gut Guide: easy to digest, soothing and full of nourishment.

SERVES 4

1.5 litres (51 fl oz/6 cups) fish Bone Broth or
    Vegetarian Broth (page 229), or store-bought stock
½ leek, white part only, halved lengthways
    & finely sliced
100 g (3½ oz) baby spinach, shredded
2 large handfuls flat-leaf (Italian) parsley leaves,
    roughly chopped
1 large handful dill, roughly chopped
sea salt & freshly ground black pepper, to taste
extra-virgin olive oil, for drizzling

Herbed Fish Balls
500 g (1 lb 2 oz) filleted skinless & boneless
    barramundi or other white fish
2 large free-range organic egg whites
½ onion, finely chopped
2 garlic cloves, finely chopped
1 small handful flat-leaf (Italian) parsley leaves,
    finely chopped
1 small handful dill, finely chopped
1 teaspoon sea salt
¼ teaspoon freshly ground white pepper

To prepare the herbed fish balls, blend the fish in a food processor until finely chopped. Transfer to a medium bowl, add the remaining ingredients, and mix well. Cover and refrigerate for 15 minutes to bind.

Using clean, wet hands, shape the fish mixture into 12 golf ball–sized balls. Place on a plate and set aside.

In a medium saucepan, bring the broth and leek to a simmer over a medium heat. Cook for 5 minutes, or until the leek softens. Reduce the heat to just below simmering, then add the fish balls. Poach for 5–7 minutes until firm and just cooked through. Add the spinach, parsley and dill and stir gently until just wilted. Season with salt and pepper.

Serve drizzled with extra-virgin olive oil.

CARLA'S TIP If you want to use chicken or vegetable broth in place of fish here, it will work just as well.

LOW-FODMAP OPTION Omit the onion and garlic and use the green part of the leek instead of the white part.

Saffron Fish Chowder

I have always found chowder super satisfying. So much so that I used to buy this soup weekly from my lovely friend Diana, who offered it on the menu of her community food co-op. It is so generous, nourishing and creamy, and the vibrant saffron does a little more than just make this soup pop. A key component in this spice – crocin – may help treat symptoms associated with digestive disorders, including inflammation. I've added sweet potato too, because it's delicious and a good source of resistant starch.

SERVES 4

500 ml (17 fl oz/2 cups) fish Bone Broth or Vegetarian
    Broth (page 229), or store-bought stock
1 medium parsnip, peeled & diced
pinch of saffron threads
½ teaspoon sweet paprika
2 tablespoons ghee or extra-virgin olive or coconut oil
1 leek, white part only, sliced into 1 cm (½ in) rounds
3 celery stalks, diced
1 medium onion, diced
2 garlic cloves, finely chopped
300 g (10½ oz, 1 medium) sweet potato, diced
200 ml (7 fl oz) coconut cream
350–400 g (12½–14 oz) skinless barramundi fillet,
    cut into bite-sized chunks
200 g (7 oz) skinless salmon fillet,
    cut into bite-sized chunks
1 red capsicum (bell pepper), diced
1 large handful flat-leaf (Italian) parsley leaves,
    coarsely chopped
sea salt & freshly ground black pepper, to taste
lemon wedges, to serve (optional)

Pour the broth into a small saucepan. Add the parsnip, saffron threads and paprika and bring to the boil. Simmer for 10 minutes, or until tender. Using a hand-held or electric blender, blend until smooth. Set aside.

Heat the ghee in a medium saucepan over a low–medium heat. Cook the leek, celery, onion and garlic for about 3 minutes until softened. Add the sweet potato and stir to combine. Gradually pour in the saffron fish broth and simmer for 10 minutes, or until the sweet potato is tender when pierced with a fork.

Add the coconut cream, barramundi, salmon and capsicum and stir to combine. Simmer for 5–7 minutes, without stirring, until the fish is just cooked and flakes easily. Add the parsley and gently stir to combine. Season with salt and pepper to taste. Serve with lemon wedges, if desired.

CARLA'S TIP As this soup is quite thick, you need to watch it attentively to ensure it doesn't burn on the bottom. Just make sure to stir it gently so as to not break up the pieces of fish.

LOW-FODMAP OPTION Use the green part of the leek instead of the white, reduce the celery to 1 stalk and swap the onion for the green part of 3 spring onions (scallions). Omit the garlic.

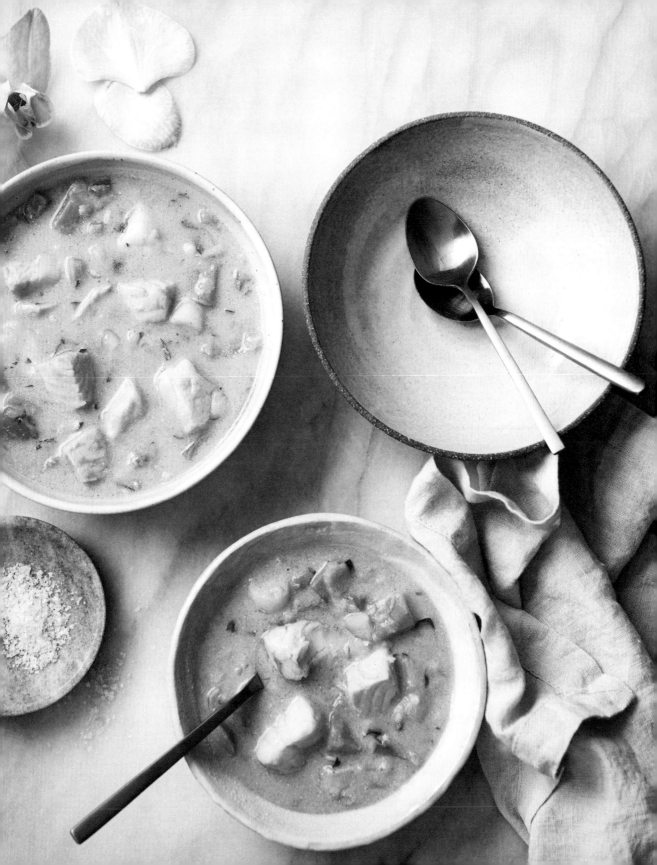

Pick-Your-Own-Herbs Oven-Baked Barramundi

Eating a simplified diet when healing the gut doesn't have to be boring, which is why I've created three herb blends you can use to create different versions of oven-baked barramundi. I've also made sure to include digestive elements such as parsley, lemon juice, dill and turmeric. Capers are also great for your tummy, as they are an excellent source of gut-healing quercetin.

SERVES 2

2 × 200 g (7 oz) skinless barramundi fillets

Parsley, Lemon & Capers
1½ tablespoons extra-virgin olive oil
finely grated zest of 1 unwaxed lemon
2 tablespoons freshly squeezed lemon juice
1 handful flat-leaf (Italian) parsley, finely chopped
¼ teaspoon each sea salt
   & freshly ground black pepper
1 tablespoon capers

Dill, Turmeric & Sea Salt
1½ tablespoons extra-virgin olive oil
1 tablespoon freshly squeezed lemon juice
1 handful dill, finely chopped
2 teaspoons ground turmeric
¼ teaspoon each sea salt &
   freshly ground black pepper

Basil, Chilli & Green Olives
1 tablespoon extra-virgin olive oil
1 tablespoon freshly squeezed lemon juice
1 handful basil, finely chopped
1 long red chilli, seeds removed, finely diced
8 green olives, pitted, finely diced
freshly ground black pepper & sea salt, to taste

CARLA'S TIP These herb mixes will work well with other varieties of fish too, so check in with your local fishmonger to see what sustainable fish is fresh that day.

Preheat the oven to 200°C (400°F/Gas Mark 6) and line a baking tray with baking paper.

Choose your herb mix and combine the ingredients in a medium bowl. Add the fish fillets and rub in the spices to coat.

Place the fish on the pre-lined tray and bake for 10–15 minutes until it is just cooked through and flakes easily. Serve with Gut-Healing Turmeric & Parsley Tabouleh (page 198) or another side of your choice.

As an alternative preparation method, you can cook the fish in parcels. It partially steams and poaches it in the delicious herb mix, making it succulent and full of flavour. Line a piece of aluminium foil (big enough to fit the fish fillets) with a piece of slightly smaller baking paper. Space the fish out on top (or make separate parcels) and cover with the herb mix. Fold to enclose, pinching the edges to form an airtight parcel. Place on a baking tray and cook at the same temperature and time as for the baked fish.

Gluten Free   Dairy Free   Stage 1 Friendly   Low FODMAP

Lemongrass & Kaffir Lime Salmon Cakes

Lemongrass and kaffir lime leaves don't just complement each other in flavour – they share a number of organic anti-inflammatory compounds shown to support healthy digestion. Salmon is a good source of vitamin B3, which is important for the metabolic functions of the digestive system. These cakes are very moreish and make a great dinner with this Asian slaw or a dollop of aioli.

SERVES 4 (Makes 12 cakes)

Salmon Cakes

800 g (1 lb 12 oz) skinless salmon fillet, pin-boned,
    cut into 1.5 cm (½ in) cubes
40 g (1½ oz/⅓ cup) arrowroot
2 free-range organic egg whites
1 lemongrass stem (white part only),
    bruised & finely diced
8 kaffir lime leaves, finely shredded
1 tablespoon fresh ginger, finely chopped
1 long red chilli, seeds removed,
    finely chopped (optional)
½ teaspoon sea salt
¼ teaspoon freshly ground black pepper
2 tablespoons extra-virgin coconut oil

Asian Slaw

250 g (9 oz) Chinese cabbage (wombok),
    finely shredded
200 g (7 oz) red cabbage, finely shredded
1 medium carrot, finely shredded
150 g (5½ oz/1½ cups) mung bean sprouts
1 handful coriander (cilantro) stems & leaves
1 handful mint
2 spring onions (scallions), green part only, finely sliced

Tamari Lime Dressing

60 ml (2 fl oz/¼ cup) freshly squeezed lime juice
1½ tablespoons tamari
1 tablespoon mirin
1 teaspoon sesame oil

To prepare the slaw, toss all ingredients in a medium bowl to combine. In a separate bowl, combine the dressing ingredients and mix well.

Add the dressing to the slaw and toss to combine.

To prepare the salmon cakes, put all ingredients except the coconut oil in a medium bowl and stir to combine.

Heat 1 tablespoon of the oil in a large frying pan over a medium–high heat. Drop a quarter cup of the salmon mixture into the pan and flatten slightly, using the back of a spatula, to form a 1.5 cm (½ in) patty. Cook for 2 minutes on each side, or until golden and just cooked through. Transfer to a plate, cover to keep warm and repeat the process with the remaining salmon mixture.

Serve the cakes with some Asian slaw.

CARLA'S TIP If you can't find kaffir lime leaves or lemongrass, substitute with finely grated lime or lemon zest. These fish cakes would also pair nicely with Lime Cream (page 190). If you're having this dish in Stage 1, eat it without slaw and serve with steamed bok choy drizzled with sesame oil instead.

Gluten Free   Dairy Free   Stage 4 Friendly   Low FODMAP

Chicken, Vegetable & Buckwheat Soup

This is one of my go-to soups, and I have small batches of it frozen for a quick and easy breakfast or lunch. It's a fabulous recipe to nourish your body with an abundance of beneficial nutrients – the soup liquid absorbs them when they leach out of the vegetables as they cook. The herbs, bitter greens and celery help stimulate digestive enzymes and are a rich source of antioxidant flavonoids that help boost microbial diversity and reduce pathogenic bacteria.

SERVES 6

150 g (5½ oz/¾ cup) buckwheat groats
splash of unpasteurised apple-cider vinegar
2 tablespoons ghee or extra-virgin olive oil
½ leek, white part only, sliced
1 medium onion, thinly sliced
1 celery stick, finely diced
3 tablespoons fresh ginger, finely chopped
3 garlic cloves, finely chopped
1 long red chilli, finely sliced (optional)
1 small handful oregano, finely chopped
1 small handful thyme, coarsely chopped
2 litres (68 fl oz/8 cups) chicken Bone Broth or
    Vegetarian Broth (page 229), or store-bought stock
400–450 g (14 oz–1 lb, about 2) organic chicken
    breasts (or cooked chickpeas, see Tip)
150 g (5½ oz/2 cups) white cabbage, shredded
3 large kale leaves, stems removed & leaves shredded
1 medium carrot, coarsely grated
1 medium zucchini (courgette), coarsely grated
2 large handfuls flat-leaf (Italian) parsley leaves,
    coarsely chopped
1 handful bitter greens, such as rocket (arugula)
    or chicory (endive)
sea salt & freshly ground black pepper, to taste

Fill a small bowl up halfway with warm water. Add the buckwheat groats and vinegar and set aside in a warm place to soak for at least 2 (and up to 6) hours. Drain and set aside.

Melt the ghee in a stockpot over a low–medium heat. Add the leek, onion, celery, ginger and garlic and cook for 3–4 minutes until softened. Add the chilli (if using), oregano and thyme and sauté for 1 minute, or until fragrant.

Pour in the broth and bring to the boil. Reduce to a simmer, then add the chicken. Cover and poach for 15 minutes, or until the chicken is just cooked through and the juices run clear when you pierce the thickest part of the breast. Transfer the chicken to a bowl and set aside for 10 minutes, or until cool enough to handle.

Add the buckwheat, cabbage, kale, carrot and zucchini to the pot and simmer for 10 minutes, or until tender.

Shred the chicken and return it to the soup. Add the parsley and bitter greens and stir to combine. Season with salt and pepper to taste.

CARLA'S TIP For a vegetarian version, swap the chicken for 300 g (10½ oz/1½ cups) cooked chickpeas – they add a nice little boost of veggie-friendly protein and a mix of soluble and insoluble fibre to feed the beneficial bacteria in your gut.

LOW-FODMAP OPTION Omit the onion and garlic. Use the green part of the leek instead of the white.

Gluten Free   Dairy-Free Option   Vegetarian Option   Stage 2 Friendly   Low-FODMAP Option

Chicken, Wombok, Asparagus & Pea Soup

When we are in harmony with our microbiome, health and wellbeing follow. A nutrient-balanced soup is one of the best ways to help make this happen. Nothing is more nourishing than a good, heart-warming chicken soup, especially when combined with a powerhouse of nutrient-rich, prebiotic greens. Leek, wombok (Chinese cabbage), asparagus, silverbeet (Swiss Chard), peas and spring onions (scallions) give this broth an anti-inflammatory and antioxidant superboost. Top it all off with the fermented goodness, and deliciousness, of Miso & Wakame Butter (page 245) for extra richness.

SERVES 4

2 tablespoons ghee or extra-virgin olive oil
1 leek, white part only, sliced
1½ tablespoons fresh ginger, finely chopped
3 garlic cloves, finely chopped
1.5 litres (51 fl oz/6 cups) chicken Bone Broth or
    Vegetarian Broth (page 229), or store-bought stock
400–450 g (14 oz–1 lb, around 2) organic
    chicken breasts
300 g (10½ oz) wombok (Chinese cabbage),
    coarsely chopped
3 leaves silverbeet with stems (Swiss chard), thinly
    sliced
160 g (5½ oz, about 1 bunch) asparagus, woody ends
    trimmed, halved lengthways
100 g (3½ oz/¾ cup) frozen peas
3 spring onions (scallions), finely sliced
sea salt & freshly ground black pepper
Miso & Wakame Butter (page 245), to serve

Melt the ghee in a medium saucepan over a low–medium heat. Cook the leek, ginger and garlic until softened, about 2 minutes. Pour in the broth and bring to the boil. Decrease the heat to a gentle simmer and add the chicken. Cover and poach for 15 minutes, or until the chicken is just cooked through and the juices run clear when you pierce the thickest part of the breast.

Transfer the chicken to a bowl and set aside for 10 minutes, or until cool enough to handle. Shred the chicken, then return it to the soup.

Add the wombok, silverbeet, asparagus, peas and spring onions. Gently simmer for 3–4 minutes until the asparagus is tender.

Season with salt and pepper and serve topped with a thin slice (approx. 0.5 cm/¼ in) of Miso & Wakame Butter.

CARLA'S TIP If you've got any of the Herb-Infused Chicken Patties (page 141) in the freezer, swap them for the chicken breasts and you've got a whole new version of this delicious soup!

Gluten Free   Dairy-Free Option   Stage 3 Friendly

Fig, Garlic & Oregano Braised Chicken

Baked chicken is my family's Sunday night dinner ritual. It's so easy, versatile and full of flavour, and nourishing for the week ahead. This simple yet delectable combination of fig, lemon, garlic and oregano has been used in Mediterranean cooking well before we knew about these ingredients' benefits for our health. Lemons are high in vitamin C, an essential nutrient for fighting inflammation, figs are a great source of fibre and garlic provides a good source of prebiotic inulin. Carvacrol, the most abundant phenol in oregano, has a bunch of benefits too, and is shown to stop the growth of several types of pathogenic gut bacteria.

SERVES 4

1.4 kg (3 lb 1 oz, or 4) organic chicken leg quarters
60 ml (2 fl oz/¼ cup) extra-virgin olive oil
125 ml (4 fl oz/½ cup) freshly squeezed lemon juice
zest of 2 unwaxed lemons
6 garlic cloves, finely chopped
1 handful oregano, coarsely chopped
sea salt & freshly ground black pepper
1 medium onion, quartered
375 ml (12½ fl oz/1½ cups) chicken Bone Broth or
    Vegetarian Broth (page 229), or store-bought stock
1 tablespoon unpasteurised apple-cider vinegar
3 ripe figs, roughly torn in half (only use if in season)
Spice-Roasted Cauliflower with Nut Butter Cream,
    Almonds & Herbs (page 195) or Green Beans,
    Sauteed Fennel, Capers & Herbs (page 199),
    to serve

Arrange the chicken in a large, deep baking dish.

In a small bowl, combine the olive oil with the lemon juice and zest, garlic and oregano. Season with salt and pepper. Pour the mixture over the chicken, rubbing it into and under the skin to coat. Cover and refrigerate for at least 1 hour, and up to 8 hours.

When ready, preheat the oven to 180°C (350°F/ Gas Mark 4).

Scatter the onion around the chicken. Pour in the bone broth and vinegar and drizzle with the remaining oil. Cook, uncovered, for 50 minutes, or until golden brown and cooked through – the juices should run clear when a fork is inserted into the thickest part of the thigh. If using figs, add them for the final 15 minutes of cooking.

Remove the chicken and figs (if using) from the baking dish. Place on a plate, cover and keep warm. Pour the liquid into a small saucepan and simmer for 3–4 minutes, or until reduced to a sauce that thinly coats the back of a spoon. Return the chicken and figs to the baking dish and coat in the sauce before serving.

Serve with Spice-Roasted Cauliflower with Nut Butter Cream, Almonds & Herbs or Green Beans, Sauteed Fennel, Capers & Herbs, or a side of your choice.

CARLA'S TIP If figs aren't in season, you can use pear instead. Simply peel, core and cut into thick slices and add to the dish with the chicken.

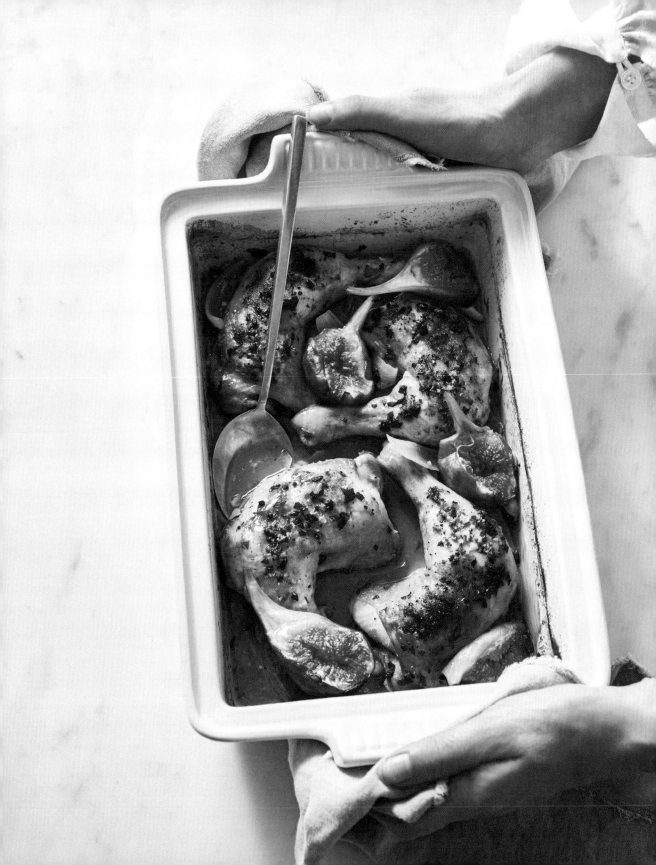

Baked Lemon Chicken with Leeks & Green Olives

When all of the flavours align in a recipe, you have a winning dish – and in this case, a healthy one. While leeks are rich in prebiotic compounds, olives contain postbiotic compounds as a result of their lactic acid fermentation. Olives also contain anti-inflammatory and antimicrobial phenolic compounds. This 'biotic' potential makes them not only great for your gut, but a winner for your metabolic and immune health too.

SERVES 4

1.5 kg (3 lb 5 oz, about 8) organic chicken thighs, skin on, bone in
80 ml (2½ oz/⅓ cup) ghee or extra-virgin olive oil
sea salt & freshly ground black pepper, to taste
2 leeks, green part only, thickly sliced into rounds
3 teaspoons fresh ginger, finely grated
2 teaspoons ground coriander
2 teaspoons ground cumin
½ teaspoon ground turmeric
750 ml (25½ fl oz/3 cups) chicken Bone Broth or Vegetarian Broth (page 229), or store-bought stock
180 g (6½ oz/1 cup) Sicilian olives
1 unwaxed lemon, cut into 8 wedges, seeds removed
2 large handfuls coriander (cilantro) leaves & stems
2 large handfuls flat-leaf (Italian) parsley leaves
50 g (1¾ oz/⅓ cup) hazelnuts, roasted, peeled & coarsely chopped
Sweet Potato Chips with Lime Cream (page 190), Green Beans, Sautéed Fennel, Capers & Herbs (page 199) or Roasted Carrot, Witlof & Toasted Walnut Salad with Orange & Umeboshi Dressing (page 196), to serve

Brine
60 g (2 oz/½ cup) sea salt
125 ml (4 fl oz/½ cup) boiling water
1 litre (34 fl oz/4 cups) chilled or iced water
60 ml (2 fl oz/¼ cup) unpasteurised apple-cider vinegar

To prepare the brine, combine the salt and boiling water in a large bowl, stirring to dissolve the salt. Add the chilled water and vinegar. Stir to combine, add the chicken, cover and refrigerate for 2 hours.

Remove the chicken from the brine and pat dry with a paper towel. Preheat the oven to 180°C (350°F/Gas Mark 4).

Heat 2 tablespoons of the ghee in a medium ovenproof stockpot or a heavy-based ovenproof saucepan with a lid over a medium–high heat. Season the chicken with salt and pepper and cook, starting skin side down, for 3–4 minutes on each side until golden. Transfer to a plate.

Reduce to a low–medium heat and add the remaining ghee to the pan. Cook the leek and ginger until soft and golden, about 2 minutes. Add the spices and cook for 30 seconds, or until fragrant. Pour in the broth and bring to the boil.

Remove the pan from the heat. Return the chicken to the pan and scatter with the olives, lemon, coriander and parsley.

Cover and bake for 40 minutes, or until the chicken juices run clear when a skewer is inserted into the thickest part of a thigh, near the bone. Remove the chicken from the pan, place on a plate and cover to keep warm.

Place the pan over a medium heat and simmer for another 3–4 minutes until the liquid is thick enough to coat the back of a spoon. Return the chicken to the pan and coat it in the sauce.

Scatter with the roasted hazelnuts and serve with some of the recommended sides.

Gluten Free   Dairy-Free Option   Stage 3 Friendly   Low FODMAP

Herb-Infused Chicken Patties

Full of aromatic herbs and spices, these moreish, savoury and spicy patties are an easy dinner paired with a salad, or a great lunchbox filler. Ginger is anti-inflammatory, and oregano and chilli are both antimicrobial. Fennel seeds help ease the symptoms associated with digestive disorders and fight the unfavourable bacteria that cause them. If you are not a big fan of chilli or you're making these for kids, reduce the amount of chilli a bit, as they do have quite a bite.

SERVES 4 (Makes 8 patties/16 small meatballs)

750 g (1 lb 11 oz) lean free-range chicken mince

2 teaspoons oregano, finely chopped

3 teaspoons fresh ginger, finely grated

1½ tablespoons nutritional yeast flakes

1 tablespoon unpasteurised apple-cider vinegar

1 tablespoon fennel seeds, lightly toasted
    & coarsely ground

1 large organic egg white

zest of 1 unwaxed lemon

1 teaspoon dried chilli flakes
    (or less, as they are spicy)

¾ teaspoon sea salt

½ teaspoon freshly ground black pepper

2 tablespoons extra-virgin olive or coconut oil

Put all ingredients except the oil in a medium bowl. Using clean hands or a wooden spoon, mix and knead the mixture until well combined.

Shape it into 8 patties or 16 meatballs. Place on a tray, cover and refrigerate for 20 minutes.

Heat 1 tablespoon of the oil in a large frying pan over a medium heat. Cook half the patties or meatballs, turning frequently, for 5–8 minutes until browned all over and just cooked through. Transfer onto a plate or clean tray and set aside. Repeat with the remaining oil and patties or meatballs.

CARLA'S TIP You can substitute other herbs in this recipe, if you like. I sometimes use marjoram instead of oregano, and it is just as delicious.

Gluten Free   Dairy Free   Stage 2 Friendly   Low FODMAP

Chicken, Flaked Almond & Sage Buckwheat 'Risotto'

This recipe comforts, satiates and is creamy and delicious. Buckwheat is a great gluten- and wheat-free grain alternative for sensitive stomachs. It is also a very good source of manganese, a mineral that is key for the production of a range of digestive enzymes. Soaking your groats for 2 to 6 hours is important to break down phytic acid, making this seed more digestible and even gentler on the gut. I've boosted this dish with vitamin E-rich almonds and woody sage, a powerful anti-inflammatory agent shown to ease the symptoms associated with poor digestion.

SERVES 4

200 g (7 oz/1 cup) buckwheat groats
splash of unpasteurised apple-cider vinegar
1.5 litres (51 fl oz/6 cups) chicken Bone Broth or
　　Vegetarian Broth (page 229), or store-bought stock
2 tablespoons ghee or extra-virgin olive oil
400–450 g (14 oz–1 lb, about 2) organic
　　chicken breasts
sea salt & freshly ground black pepper, to taste
15 g (½ oz/⅓ cup) nutritional yeast flakes
zest of 1 unwaxed lemon
60 ml (2 fl oz/¼ cup) freshly squeezed lemon juice

Fried Almonds & Sage
80 ml (2½ fl oz/⅓ cup) ghee or extra-virgin olive oil
50 g (1¾ oz) flaked almonds
4 handfuls sage leaves

CARLA'S TIP For a variation, try adding some roasted pumpkin (squash) or bitter greens such as dandelion or chickory to your 'risotto'.

Fill a small bowl halfway with warm water. Add the buckwheat groats and vinegar and set aside in a warm place to soak for at least 2 (and up to 6) hours. Drain and rinse.

Preheat the oven at 180°C (350°F/Gas Mark 4).

Combine the buckwheat groats and broth in a medium wide-based saucepan and place over a medium heat. Simmer, stirring occasionally, for 20–25 minutes, or until the buckwheat has absorbed almost all of the liquid and is tender and creamy, but still has a slight bite.

Meanwhile, heat the ghee in a medium ovenproof frying pan over a medium–high heat. Season the chicken breasts with salt and pepper. Cook, smooth-side down, for 3 minutes, or until golden brown. Flip the breasts and finish cooking in the oven for 10–15 minutes until golden brown and just cooked through (the juices should run clear when pierced with a knife). Transfer onto a plate, cover loosely with foil and rest for 5 minutes.

To prepare the almonds and sage, heat the ghee in a small frying pan over a medium–high heat. Fry them, tossing occasionally, for 3 minutes, or until the almonds turn golden brown and the sage is crisp. Remove from the heat and set aside.

Add the yeast flakes, lemon zest and juice to the saucepan with the risotto and stir to combine.

Slice the chicken breasts and serve on top of the risotto with some fried almonds and sage. Drizzle with the remaining ghee from the pan.

　　Gluten Free　　Dairy-Free Option　　Stage 4 Friendly　　Low FODMAP

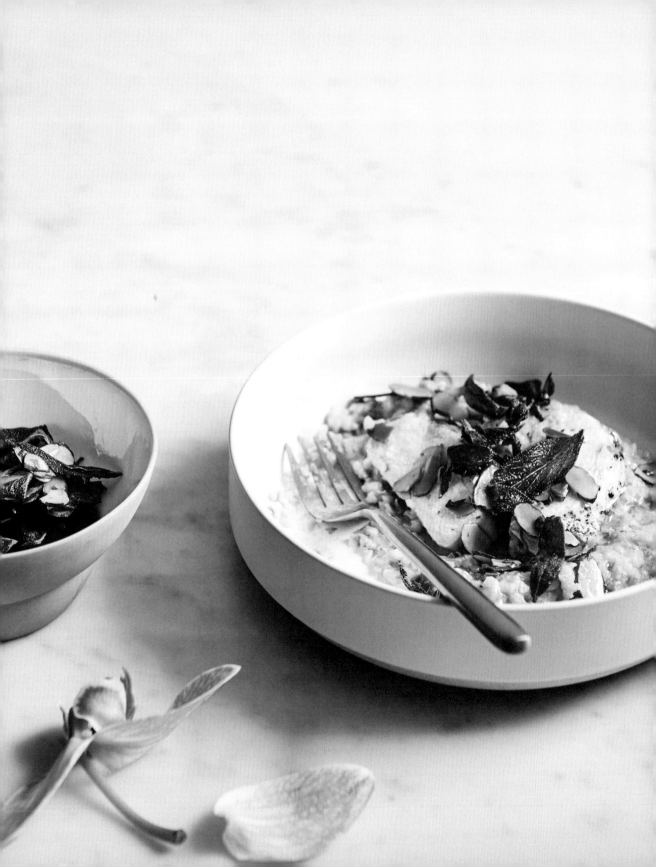

Spiced Chicken, Three Ways

Variety is the spice of life. Take one piece of chicken and experience a different culinary journey every time. These interesting, delicious spice mixes will keep your tastebuds inspired during your Stage 1 diet. I prefer to use chicken thighs, as I find breasts too dry, but it is up to you. Spiced drumsticks and wings also make great afternoon snacks. If you want a vegetarian or vegan option, try sprinkling these spice mixes over wedges of pumpkin, roasted sweet potatoes or other roasted vegetables.

SERVES 2

250–300 g (9–10½ oz, about 2) organic chicken
    thighs (boneless) or breasts
coconut, ghee or extra-virgin olive oil, for frying

Piri Piri Spice Mix
2 teaspoons smoked paprika
½ teaspoon cayenne pepper
a few grinds of sea salt &
    freshly ground black pepper
2 teaspoons dried oregano
zest of 1 unwaxed lemon

Middle Eastern Spice Mix
1 teaspoon ground cinnamon
1 teaspoon ground nutmeg
1 teaspoon ground coriander
1 teaspoon ground cumin
1 teaspoon smoked paprika
¼ teaspoon each sea salt &
    freshly ground black pepper

Greek Herb & Spice Mix
1 teaspoon dried basil
1 teaspoon dried oregano
1 teaspoon dried parsley
2 teaspoons ground cumin
zest of 1 unwaxed lemon
¼ teaspoon each sea salt &
    freshly ground black pepper

In a medium bowl, combine the ingredients of the spice mix of your choice. Add the chicken and rub in the spice mix to coat.

Pour coconut oil into a medium frying pan to a depth of about 1 cm (½ in). Place over a medium–high heat. Add the chicken and fry for 5–6 minutes on each side until golden and cooked through. Cooking time will vary depending on the thickness of your chicken. To check for doneness, slice into the thickest part of the thigh or breast.

CARLA'S TIP Premake your spices in bulk and store them in sterilised jars to have on hand for a quick and easy midweek timesaver. For a delicious alternative to frying, turn the spice mixes into pastes by adding 1 tablespoon of extra-virgin olive oil to your chosen mix, plus an additional 1 tablespoon of lemon juice to the Greek Herb & Spice Mix. Line a piece of aluminium foil (big enough to fit the chicken) with a piece of slightly smaller baking paper. Space the chicken out on top and spread with the spice mix to coat. Fold to enclose, pinching the edges to form an airtight parcel. Place on a baking tray and cook at 200°C (400°F/Gas Mark 6) for 5 minutes. Remove from the oven and set aside to rest for 5 minutes. Serve with steamed greens.

Vietnamese-Style Chicken Lettuce Cups

Fresh and brimming with flavour, these cups of deliciousness make a healthy, light lunch or dinner and are a great way to get the family 'hands on' by assembling their own cups. Store-bought hoisin sauces contain upwards of 5 g (¼ oz) sugar per tablespoon, and a host of artificial ingredients (namely MSG), which is why I've come up with a homemade version minus the nasties. I've included manuka honey for its antibacterial benefits, gut-healthy miso and apple-cider vinegar for digestive support, and a hint of garlic and ginger to fight inflammation.

SERVES 4 (Makes 8 lettuce cups)

1 large head iceberg lettuce

2 tablespoons extra-virgin coconut oil

1 red capsicum (bell pepper), finely sliced lengthways

2 tablespoons fresh ginger, finely chopped

1 garlic clove, finely chopped

500 g (1 lb 2 oz) chicken mince

1½ tablespoons freshly squeezed lime juice

3 spring onions (scallions), white part only, finely sliced

2 large handfuls bean shoots

2 large handfuls coriander (cilantro), stems & leaves

1 large handful Vietnamese mint

1 large handful Vietnamese basil

2 tablespoons white sesame seeds

Hoisin Sauce

3 Medjool dates, pitted & coarsely chopped

80 ml (2½ fl oz/⅓ cup) just boiled water

90 g (3 oz/⅓ cup) red miso paste

1 tablespoon unpasteurised apple-cider vinegar

1 tablespoon manuka honey

2 teaspoons tamari

1 garlic clove

2 teaspoons fresh ginger, coarsely chopped

1½ teaspoons Chinese five-spice

Remove 8 crisp centre leaves from the iceberg head and put them in a bowl of ice water.

To prepare the hoisin sauce, soak the dates in the boiling water for 10 minutes, or until softened. Blitz them, their soaking liquid and all remaining ingredients in a high-speed blender until smooth. Transfer to a small bowl and set aside.

Heat the oil in a large frying pan or wok over a high heat. Stir-fry the capsicum, ginger and garlic for 1 minute, or until softened. Add the chicken mince and cook, using a wooden spoon to break up any big lumps, for 3–4 minutes, or until browned. Turn the heat down to medium, then add 125 ml (4 fl oz/½ cup) hoisin sauce and the lime juice. Bring to a simmer, stirring to combine.

Add the spring onion, bean shoots, coriander, mint, basil and sesame seeds and stir to combine. Remove the pan from the heat.

Remove the lettuce cups from the ice water and shake dry. Working with one lettuce leaf at a time, spoon approximately one-third of a cup of chicken filling into the centre. Serve as a cup, or fold in the sides and roll up to form a log-shaped parcel.

CARLA'S TIP This hoisin sauce can be made in a double batch and stored in an airtight container in the refrigerator for up to 3 weeks. A spoonful adds a great flavour twist to soups, tempeh or vegetable stir-fry, and is also served with steamed chicken.

Gluten Free   Dairy Free   Stage 3 Friendly

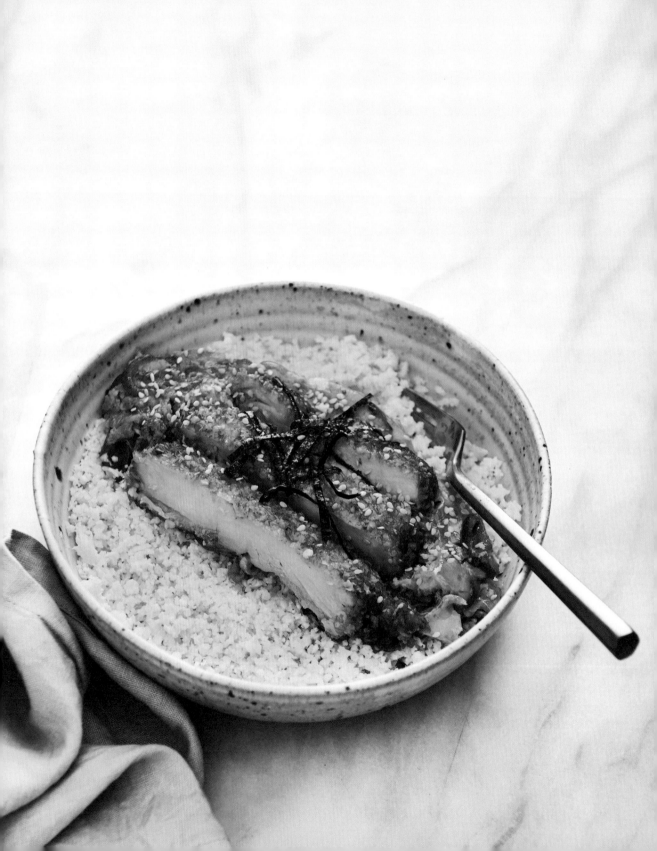

Chicken Katsu Don

I love chicken katsu, but my other half (my microbiome) doesn't. Here is a healthier and even yummier version that I eat occasionally (because it is fried). When you put chicken katsu into dashi broth, and egg on a bed of 'rice', you create chicken katsu don. Dashi is a traditional Japanese stock used as a base for miso soup, and primarily stems from two ingredients – kombu and katsuobushi. Kombu is a type of seaweed that is great at helping break down the heavy starches found in legumes and beans due to its amino acid composition. It also contains the natural polysaccharide fucoidan, which studies have shown can help reduce gastritis and gastric ulcers and protect the stomach's mucosal lining.

SERVES 4

6 free-range organic eggs, lightly beaten
1 tablespoon ghee or extra-virgin olive oil
320 g (11½ oz) silverbeet (Swiss chard) leaves, shredded
1½ tablespoons freshly squeezed lemon juice
1 quantity Cauliflower Rice (page 240), to serve
3 spring onions (scallions), white part only, finely sliced
2 nori sheets, toasted, thinly cut into strips

Dashi Broth
1 tablespoon ghee or extra-virgin olive oil
1 medium onion, halved & sliced
250 ml (8 ½ fl oz/1 cup) instant dashi stock
60 ml (2 fl oz/¼ cup) tamari
60 ml (2 fl oz/¼ cup) mirin

Chicken Katsu
400–450 g (14 oz–1 lb, about 2) organic skinless chicken breasts
100 g (3½ oz/1 cup) quinoa flakes
75 g (2¾ oz/½ cup) white sesame seeds
30 g (1 oz/¼ cup) arrowroot
1 free-range organic egg, beaten with a splash of drinking coconut milk or other nut-based milk
coconut oil, for shallow frying

CARLA'S TIP If you're looking for a vegetarian alternative, swap chicken for tempeh or firm tofu.

LOW-FODMAP OPTION Swap the Cauliflower Rice for quinoa, buckwheat or white basmati rice. Use the green part of the spring onions instead of the white. Halve the amount of sesame seeds and omit the onion.

Recipe continues >

Gluten Free   Dairy-Free Option   Vegetarian Option   Stage 4 Friendly   Low-FODMAP Option

To make the chicken katsu, place the chicken breasts, smooth side down, on a clean chopping board. Slice the thickest part of the breast in half crossways, leaving it still intact at the edge, and fold it open like a book. Cover with baking paper and lightly pound with a mallet or a rolling pin to a thickness of approximately 1 cm (½ in).

In a medium bowl, combine the quinoa flakes and sesame seeds. Pour the arrowroot and egg wash into separate bowls. Coat the chicken with some arrowroot, shaking off any excess, then dip into the egg wash. Coat with the quinoa and sesame mixture, pressing onto the chicken to secure.

To prepare the dashi broth, melt the ghee in a large frying pan with a lid over a low–medium heat. Add the onion and sauté for 5 minutes, or until softened and golden brown. Pour in the dashi stock, tamari and mirin and bring to a simmer. Reduce the heat to low and cover to keep warm.

Pour coconut oil in a large frying pan to a depth of 2 cm (¾ in). Heat the oil over a medium heat until a quinoa flake dropped in floats straight back to the surface, bubbling and browning. Fry the chicken for 3–4 minutes on each side until crisp, golden brown and just cooked through. Transfer onto paper towel to drain, then cut crossways into thick slices.

Arrange the sliced katsu on top of the onions and dashi broth. Pour the egg mixture over the top. Cover and cook for 3–4 minutes until the egg has set but is still wet.

Meanwhile, place a clean frying pan over a low–medium heat. Melt the ghee, then add the silverbeet and lemon juice and cook until just wilted.

To serve, divide the cauliflower rice and silverbeet evenly among serving bowls. Arrange the onion, chicken katsu and egg mixture on top, pouring on any remaining dashi broth. Scatter with spring onions and top with nori strips.

Swedish Meatballs with Braised Red Cabbage

Who doesn't love a Swedish meatball? Although chicken livers might not be the first ingredient that comes to mind when making them, they add the most delicious depth of flavour. Apart from being impressively high in vitamin B12, they are also a great source of L-glutamine that, alongside the red cabbage, helps strengthen the gut lining.

SERVES 4 (makes approx. 16 meatballs)

½ medium onion, grated

250 g (9 oz) grass-fed beef mince

150 g (5½ oz) free-range pork mince

50 g (1¾ oz) organic chicken livers, finely chopped (they really must be organic)

100 g (3½ oz/1 cup) ground almonds

1 free-range organic egg

1 teaspoon sea salt

½ teaspoon freshly ground black pepper

½ teaspoon ground allspice

½ teaspoon ground nutmeg

extra-virgin olive oil, for frying

1 large handful flat-leaf (Italian) parsley leaves, coarsely chopped, to serve

Braised Red Cabbage

1 tablespoon extra-virgin olive or coconut oil

1 small onion, sliced

¼ teaspoon caraway seeds

¼ medium red cabbage, shredded

1 medium green apple, quartered, cored & sliced

60 ml (2 fl oz/¼ cup) water

1½ tablespoons unpasteurised apple-cider vinegar

Sauce

1 litre (34 fl oz/4 cups) beef or chicken Bone Broth or Vegetarian Broth (page 229), or store-bought stock

6 thyme sprigs

180 ml (6 fl oz/¾ cup) coconut cream

1½ tablespoons freshly squeezed lemon juice

2 tablespoons water

40 g (1½ oz/⅓ cup) arrowroot

2 teaspoons tamari

2 teaspoons unpasteurised apple-cider vinegar

sea salt & freshly ground black pepper, to taste

CARLA'S TIP I like to pair this dish with Cauliflower Rice (page 240) to soak up the delicious juices.

LOW-FODMAP OPTION Make the meatballs without the onion and pair them with Carrot Noodles (page 240) or Gut-Healing Turmeric & Parsley Tabouleh (page 198) instead of the braised cabbage. Omit the sauce.

Recipe continues >

Gluten Free   Dairy Free   Stage 3 Friendly   Low-FODMAP Option

To make the meatballs, combine all ingredients except the oil and parsley in a medium bowl with clean, wet hands. Shape the mixture into 16 golf ball-sized balls and arrange on a tray. Cover and refrigerate for 20 minutes.

Add enough oil to coat the base of a large frying pan and place it over a medium-high heat. Cook the meatballs in batches, turning frequently, for 4–5 minutes until browned all over. Transfer onto a clean plate or tray and set aside.

To make the braised red cabbage, heat the oil in a medium saucepan over a low-medium heat. Sauté the onion and caraway seeds until fragrant, about 2 minutes. Add the cabbage and apple and stir to combine. Pour in the water and vinegar. Cover and simmer, stirring occasionally, for 20 minutes, or until the cabbage is tender and the liquid is almost completely reduced. Set aside.

To make the sauce, pour the broth into the pan used to cook the meatballs. Bring to the boil and, using a wooden spoon, scrape off any bits stuck to the bottom. Add the thyme and simmer for 10–15 minutes until the broth has reduced by half. Pour in the coconut cream and bring to a simmer.

While the broth is reducing, combine the lemon juice, water, arrowroot, tamari and apple-cider vinegar in a small bowl. Gradually pour the mixture into the hot stock, whisking continuously. Simmer for a further 2 minutes, or until the sauce is thick enough to coat the back of a spoon. Remove the thyme and season with salt and pepper.

Return the meatballs to the sauce, stir to coat and cook at a gentle simmer for 4–5 minutes until cooked through. The meatballs will firm up as they cook; break one in half to check for doneness. Once ready, scatter with parsley and serve with braised cabbage and your choice of sides.

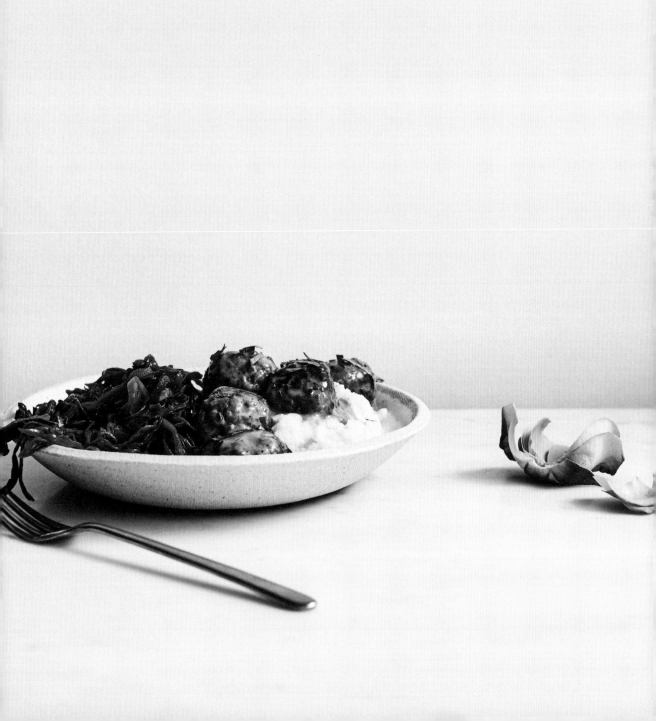

Spiced Middle Eastern Lamb Koftas

Middle Eastern cuisine is one of my favourites; I really enjoy cooking with the array of aromatic herbs and spices. Here, I've used cumin and coriander, which contain compounds that aid digestion, and mint, which acts as an anti-inflammatory. Chilli adds a nice kick from a natural chemical called capsaicin, which a study has shown inhibits the bacteria that cause ulcers.

SERVES 4 (Makes 8 koftas)

500 g (1 lb 2 oz) organic lamb mince
1 small red onion, finely diced
1 large handful flat-leaf (Italian) parsley leaves,
    coarsely chopped
1 large handful mint, coarsely chopped
2 garlic cloves, finely chopped
½ long red chilli, finely chopped
2 teaspoons ground cumin
2 teaspoons ground coriander
½ teaspoon ground cinnamon
½ teaspoon each sea salt &
    freshly ground black pepper
2 tablespoons extra-virgin olive oil,
    coconut oil or ghee

In a large bowl, combine all ingredients except the oil and mix thoroughly with clean hands.

Shape the mixture into 8 cm long (3¼ in, approx. ¼ cup each) sausages. Flatten lightly and place on a tray. Cover and refrigerate for 20 minutes, or until firm.

Preheat a large frying pan over a medium heat. Brush the koftas with oil. Cook, turning once, for 8–10 minutes, or until just cooked through. Transfer the koftas to a tray, cover with foil and allow to rest for 5 minutes.

CARLA'S TIP Lamb koftas and tabouleh marry so well together. From Stage 3, pair this dish with the Broccoli & Asparagus Tabouleh (page 200).

LOW-FODMAP OPTION Swap the onion for the green part of 2 spring onions (scallions) and omit the garlic. Serve with Gut-Healing Turmeric & Parsley Tabouleh (page 198).

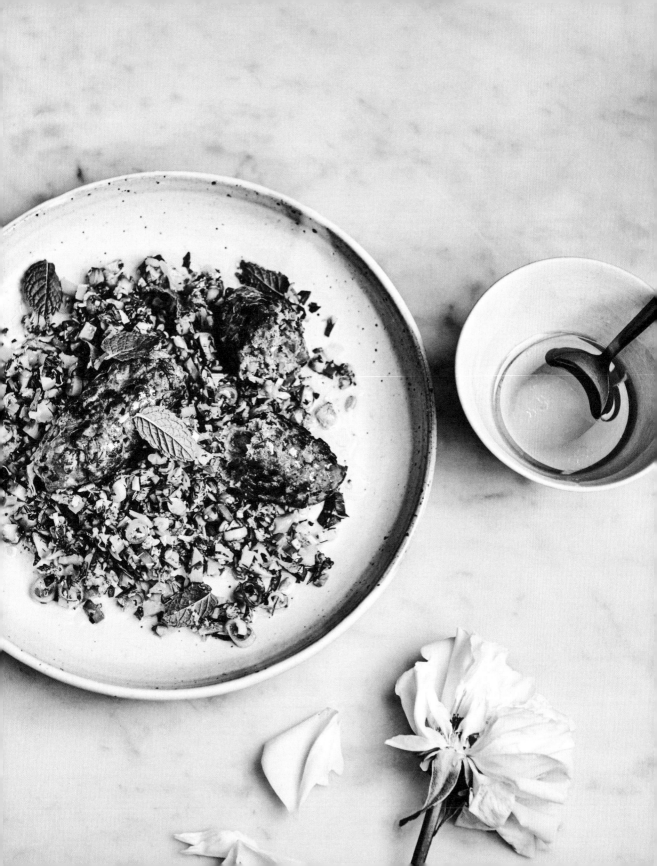

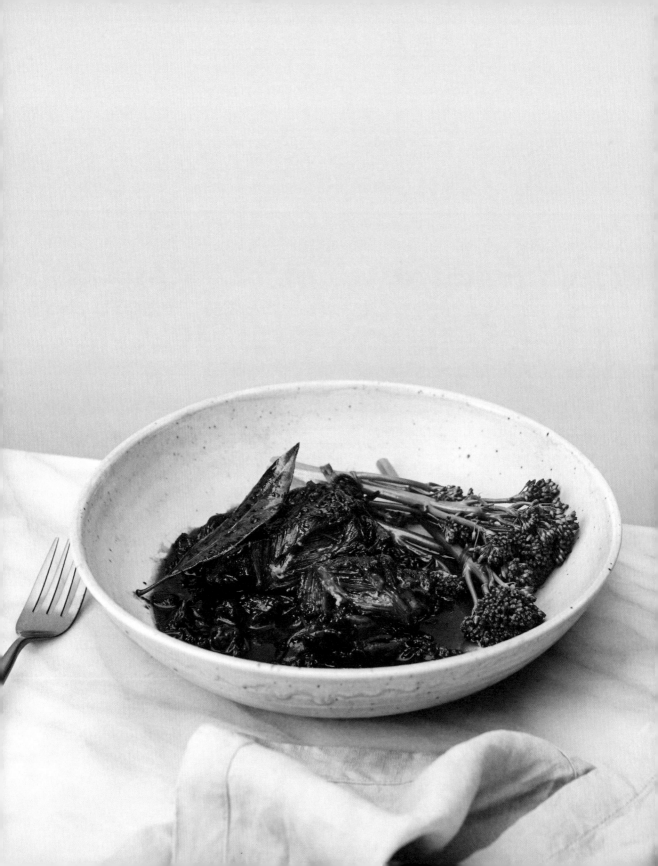

Slow-Cooked Beef Cheek
with Onions & Raisins

Generous in flavour and texture, this sticky-sweet recipe showcases why slow-cooking meat is better for your tastebuds and kinder to your gut. Slow-cooking is a great way to break down those usually hard-to-digest red meats, and allows flavours to fully develop. Always opt for grass-fed meat, as it is rich in good fats such as conjugated linoleic acid, which studies show are anti-inflammatory. It's also rich in bioavailable nutrients such as vitamins D, E, K2 and pro-vitamin A. I've added apple-cider vinegar to help stimulate the production of hydrochloric acid in the stomach, essential for proper digestion.

SERVES 4–6

2 tablespoons extra-virgin olive or coconut oil

1 tablespoon ghee

1–1.25 kg (2 lb 3 oz–2 lb 12 oz, approx. 4) beef cheeks,
    or beef blade steak/brisket cut into quarters

sea salt & freshly ground black pepper, to taste

2 medium onions, halved & sliced

2 garlic cloves, finely chopped

2 tablespoons raisins

60 ml (2 fl oz/¼ cup) unpasteurised
    apple-cider vinegar

1 litre (34 fl oz/4 cups) beef Bone Broth or Vegetarian
    Broth (page 229), or store-bought stock

6 thyme sprigs

2 rosemary stalks

2 bay leaves

Preheat the oven to 160°C (320°F/Gas Mark 3).

Heat the oil and ghee in a medium ovenproof stockpot or a heavy-based ovenproof saucepan with a lid over a medium–high heat. Season the beef with salt and pepper and cook for 3–4 minutes on each side until browned all over. Transfer to a large plate and set aside.

Add the onion and garlic to the pan and cook for 2–3 minutes until softened. Add the raisins and stir to combine. Pour in the vinegar and simmer for 1 minute, then pour in the broth and bring to the boil. Remove the pan from the heat and return the beef to it. Scatter the stew with the herbs, cover and cook in the oven for 3–3½ hours until the meat is tender and can easily be pulled apart with a fork.

If the liquid in the pan has not quite reduced enough to make a sauce, transfer the beef to a plate and cover to keep warm. Set the pan over a medium heat and simmer the liquid until it reduces enough to coat the back of a spoon. Discard the thyme, rosemary and bay leaves. Shred the beef into large chunks and return it to the pan if required. Stir and serve.

CARLA'S TIP I like to serve this dish with Sweet Potato Chips with Lime Cream (page 190) and some simple steamed greens. Remember to always have more vegetables than meat on your plate!

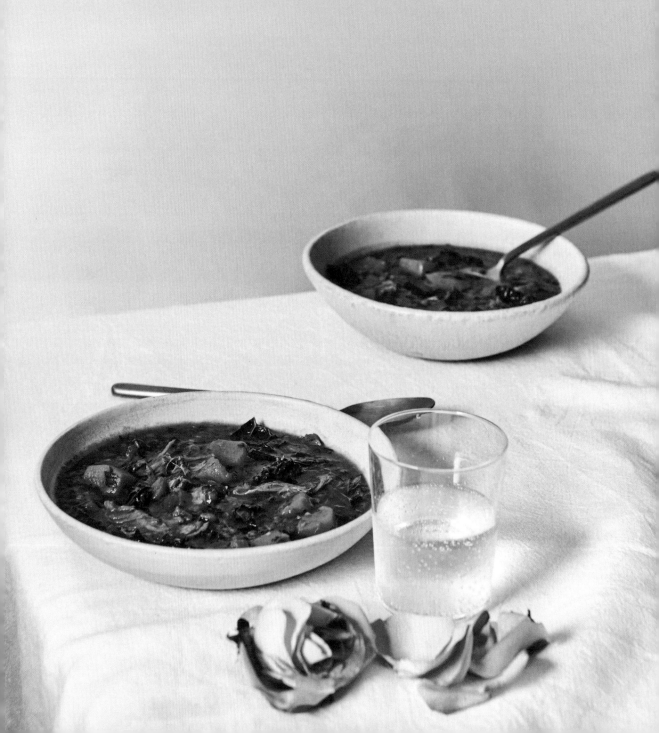

Harira Lamb Shank Soup

If you desire a soup with heart, this is it: rich in depth of flavour, texture, colour and nutrition. Lentils are a good source of protein and fibre that help balance blood sugar levels as well as nourish our belly. They are even better when used in soups, as the liquid ensures that the soluble fibre found in legumes moves easily through your system. They're also a great source of resistant starch, which helps to produce short-chain fatty acids to fight inflammation. I've opted for lamb shanks in this recipe to ensure you don't miss out on all of the gelatinous benefits of those nutrient-dense, flavourful bones.

SERVES 6

200 g (7 oz/1 cup) dried puy lentils, thoroughly rinsed
splash of unpasteurised apple-cider vinegar
60 ml (2 fl oz/¼ cup) ghee or extra-virgin olive oil
1 kg (2 lb 3 oz, about 2) lamb shanks
sea salt & freshly ground black pepper
1 large onion, diced
2 celery stalks, diced
1 medium carrot, diced
5 garlic cloves, finely chopped
2½ tablespoons fresh ginger, finely chopped
1 cinnamon stick
1½ teaspoons ground turmeric
2 teaspoons ground cumin
1 teaspoon ground coriander
½ teaspoon ground nutmeg

1.5 litres (51 fl oz/6 cups) chicken Bone Broth or Vegetarian Broth (page 229), or store-bought stock
400 g (14 oz) tinned crushed tomatoes
1 large strip kombu, rinsed
300 g (10½ oz) sweet potato, diced
4 large leaves silverbeet (Swiss chard), with stems, coarsely chopped
2 handfuls coriander (cilantro) leaves, coarsely chopped
2 handfuls flat-leaf (Italian) parsley, coarsely chopped
extra-virgin olive oil, to serve

Tedouira
30 g (1 oz/¼ cup) arrowroot
80 ml (2½ fl oz/⅓ cup) water
2 tablespoons tomato paste

CARLA'S TIP The leftovers from this soup can be simmered down and used as a 'ragu' over Buckwheat Pasta (page 233).

LOW-FODMAP OPTION Substitute 275 g (9½ oz/1 cup) rinsed and drained tinned lentils for the dried puy lentils, and add them to the soup at the end with the tedouira. Substitute the green part of 1 leek for the onion. Omit the garlic and reduce the celery to 1 stalk.

Recipe continues >

Pre-soak the lentils in a large bowl full of warm water with a splash of apple-cider vinegar for at least 7 hours (or overnight). Drain, rinse and change the water and apple-cider vinegar 1–2 times over the soaking period. Drain and set aside.

Heat the ghee in a large, heavy-based saucepan over a medium–high heat. Season the lamb shanks with salt and pepper. Cook, turning occasionally, for 5–7 minutes until browned all over. Transfer the shanks to a plate. In the same pan, cook the onion, celery, carrot, garlic and ginger until softened. Add the spices and cook for 30 seconds, or until fragrant.

Pour in the broth and tomatoes. Return the shanks to the pan and bring to the boil. Reduce to a simmer, add the kombu and cover and cook for 2 hours, or until the meat is becoming tender and starting to pull away from the bone. Add the pre-soaked lentils and sweet potato and simmer,

covered, for a further 25–30 minutes, or until the lentils and sweet potato are tender and the meat is falling off the bone.

Remove and discard the kombu. Remove the bones and meat from the pan and transfer to a large bowl. Set aside for 15 minutes, or until cool enough to handle. Using forks or clean hands, shred the lamb into small chunks and return it to the soup. Add the silverbeet and stir to combine.

To prepare the tedouira, stir all ingredients in a small bowl to make a smooth paste. Pour into the hot soup and stir to combine. Bring the soup back to a simmer and cook, stirring occasionally, for 5 minutes, or until thickened slightly. Add almost all of the coriander and parsley, reserving a little for garnish, and stir to combine. Season the soup with salt and pepper.

Serve drizzled with extra-virgin olive oil and scattered with the remaining herbs.

Indian-Spiced Sweet Potato & Lentil Cakes

These addictive spiced cakes can be prepared for dinner and are also great as a lunch box snack. Apart from being high in fibre, sweet potatoes and lentils are good sources of inflammation-fighting resistant starch and vitamin B5 (which helps maintain a healthy digestive tract). The pervading spice in this recipe is cumin, which adds such a beautiful, flavoursome note to any recipe. Studies show that it may help relieve some of the uncomfortable symptoms associated with irritable bowel syndrome.

SERVES 4 (Makes 8 cakes)

850 g (1 lb 14 oz/approx. 2 medium) sweet potatoes, peeled & cut into 3 cm (1¼ in) chunks
60 ml (2 fl oz/¼ cup) ghee or extra-virgin coconut oil, plus extra for roasting the potatoes
375 ml (12½ fl oz/1½ cups) water
110 g (4 oz/½ cup) dried red lentils, thoroughly rinsed
3 shallots, finely chopped
1½ tablespoons fresh ginger, finely chopped
2 garlic cloves, finely chopped
1 red bird's eye chilli, de-seeded, finely chopped
3 teaspoons ground cumin
1½ teaspoons ground turmeric
1½ teaspoons ground coriander
¼ teaspoon cayenne pepper (optional)
3 tablespoons arrowroot
1 tablespoon freshly squeezed lemon juice
2 large handfuls coriander (cilantro) stems & leaves, coarsely chopped
sea salt & freshly ground black pepper, to taste

Cucumber raita

250 g (9 oz/1 cup) sheep's or goat's yoghurt or coconut yoghurt
½ Lebanese (short) cucumber, cut in half lengthways, seeds scooped & grated
1 tablespoon freshly squeezed lemon juice
sea salt, to taste

CARLA'S TIP I like to serve these cakes with blanched beans and spinach dressed with extra-virgin olive oil and lemon juice. They are also delicious wrapped in Turmeric Roti (page 234) along with the raita and some fresh bitter greens.

Recipe continues >

Preheat the oven to 200°C (400°F/Gas Mark 6).

Arrange the sweet potatoes in a medium roasting tray and drizzle with some ghee. Roast for 30 minutes, or until tender.

Meanwhile, put the water and lentils in a small saucepan and bring to the boil. Reduce to a gentle simmer for 10–15 minutes, stirring occasionally to prevent the lentils from sticking, until all of the water has been absorbed and the mixture resembles a thick porridge. Set aside.

Heat 1 tablespoon of the ghee in a small frying pan. Cook the shallots, ginger, garlic and chilli until softened. Add the spices and cook for 30 seconds, or until fragrant. Transfer everything, including the roasted sweet potatoes, cooked lentils, 1 tablespoon of the arrowroot and lemon juice, to a medium bowl. Using a potato masher, mash and stir to combine, leaving some chunky bits of sweet potato. Add the coriander, season with salt and pepper and stir to combine.

Using your hands, shape the mixture into 8 cakes, approximately 7 cm (2¾ in) in diameter. Refrigerate for about 15 minutes to firm up, then lightly dust with the remaining arrowroot to coat.

Heat the remaining ghee in a large frying pan over a low–medium heat. Cook the cakes for 3–4 minutes on each side until golden brown and heated through. Set aside on a plate lined with a paper towel and cover to keep warm.

To make the cucumber raita, combine all ingredients in a bowl and stir to combine. Serve with the cakes.

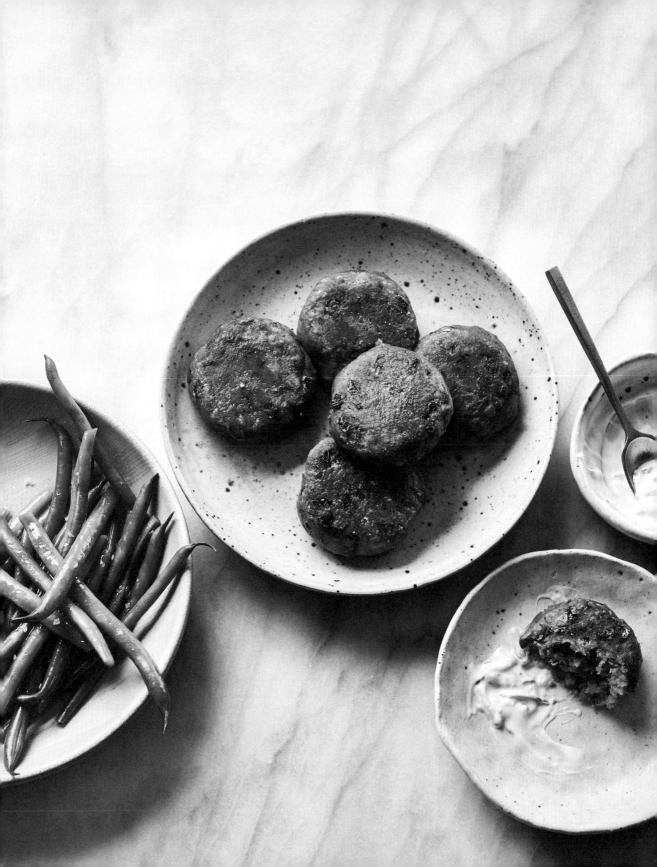

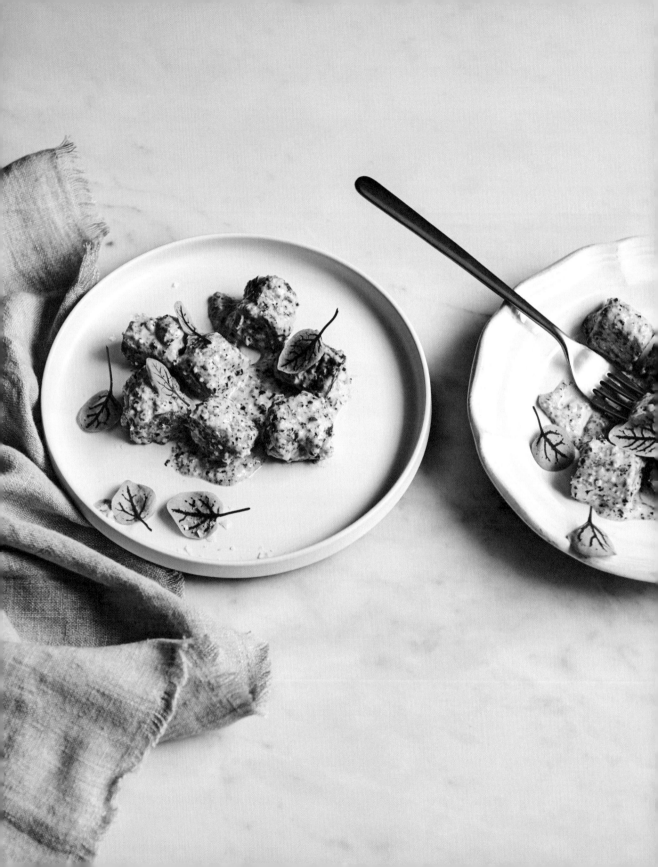

Pan-Fried Cauliflower Gnocchi with Creamy Pesto Sauce

Traditional gnocchi is delicious, but can also feel a little like heavy gut luggage. That's why I came up with a lighter, gluten-free and fibre-rich alternative that is even more flavoursome than the original. I use versatile cauliflower instead of potato and pair it with Pumpkin Seed & Herb Pesto (page 244) – a great way to add a dose of manganese and zinc, which help promote digestive enzyme function. I adore these little parcels of loveliness with pesto, but adding coconut and nut milk gives you something a little richer and creamier.

SERVES 2–3

400 g (14 oz/about ½ small) cauliflower stalk & florets, broken into large pieces
50 g (1¾ oz/½ cup) ground almonds
2 tablespoons arrowroot, plus additional for rolling
15 g (½ oz/⅓ cup) nutritional yeast flakes
1 free-range organic egg white (optional)
1 teaspoon psyllium husk
½ teaspoon sea salt
2 tablespoons ghee or extra-virgin olive oil

Creamy Pesto Sauce
125 ml (4 fl oz/½ cup) tinned coconut milk
125 ml (4 fl oz/½ cup) almond milk
90 g (3 oz/⅓ cup) Pumpkin Seed & Herb Pesto (page 244)
fresh basil, finely shredded, or micro herbs (optional), to serve
freshly ground black pepper, to serve

Steam the cauliflower for 10 minutes, or until tender. Transfer to a food processor and blend until finely chopped. Put in a medium bowl and add all remaining ingredients except the ghee. Stir to combine.

Line a baking tray with baking paper. Dust a clean kitchen bench, and your hands, with some arrowroot.

Divide the gnocchi mixture into quarters. Using your hands, gently roll one quarter at a time into 2 cm (¾ in) thick logs. Dip a small sharp knife in some arrowroot and cut each log into 2 cm (¾ in) pieces. Gently squeeze each piece in the centre to give it the classic gnocchi shape, then transfer to the prepared tray.

Melt the ghee in a large frying pan over a medium heat. Cook the gnocchi in batches for 1–2 minutes on each side until golden brown. Transfer to a plate and set aside.

To prepare the creamy pesto sauce, pour the coconut and almond milk into a frying pan and simmer over a medium heat for 2–3 minutes until reduced a bit and slightly thicker. Add the Pumpkin Seed & Herb Pesto, stirring to combine, and heat through. Add the gnocchi to the pan and ladle with sauce to coat.

Serve the gnocchi in shallow serving bowls scattered with shredded basil and topped with freshly ground black pepper.

CARLA'S TIP Due to its high soluble fibre content, psyllium husk is a great binding agent when mixed with water, helping the gnocchi maintain their fluffy, pillow-like shape. Some people find psyllium husk helpful for relieving constipation, while others find it harsh on their digestive system. I like to use it in small quantities, and usually as a binder.

Gluten Free   Dairy-Free Option   Vegetarian   Vegan Option   Stage 4 Friendly

Anise-Roasted Pumpkin Agnolotti with Walnuts, Sage & Browned Butter

This beautiful recipe may look delicate, but it boasts delicious, robust flavours that marry so well together. Star anise adds a sweet licorice note to this dish, but it also has powerful antibacterial properties. A study published in the Journal of Medicinal Food *suggests that it might have an inhibitory effect on almost 70 strains of antibiotic-resistant bacteria. Paired with the earthy-sweet flavours of gut-loving pumpkin and buckwheat, and the digestive cleansing properties of radicchio, this is sure to be a regular in your cooking repertoire.*

SERVES 4

1 quantity Buckwheat Pasta (page 233),
      prepared according to agnolotti instructions;
      cut into 40 pasta discs
1 free-range organic egg white, lightly beaten
300 g (10½ oz) salted cultured butter
60 g (2 oz/½ cup) walnuts, coarsely chopped
2 large handfuls sage leaves
100 g (3½ oz) radicchio leaves, coarsely torn
freshly ground black pepper, to serve

Filling
2 tablespoons ghee or extra-virgin olive oil
2 shallots, finely chopped
1 garlic clove, finely chopped
500 g (1 lb 2 oz) butternut pumpkin (squash),
      de-seeded & cut into 5 cm (2 in) chunks
2 tablespoons water
4 star anise
sea salt & freshly ground black pepper, to taste

To make the filling, heat the oil in a medium saucepan over a low–medium heat. Cook the shallots and garlic until softened, about 2 minutes. Add the pumpkin, water and star anise. Cover and cook, stirring occasionally, for 15 minutes, or until very tender. Discard the star anise. Transfer the pumpkin mixture to a food processor and blend until smooth. Season with salt and pepper.

Spoon 2 teaspoons of the filling into the centre of the prepared agnolotti discs. Brush around the edge with egg white. Fold the discs in half to enclose the filling, pressing around the joined edges to remove any air pockets and to seal.

Bring a large saucepan of salted water to the boil. Cook the agnolotti for 3–4 minutes until just tender or al dente. Drain and set aside.

Melt the butter in a medium frying pan over a medium heat. Add the walnuts and sage and cook until the butter begins to turn light brown and the sage and walnuts are golden and crisp. Add the radicchio and toss until wilted.

To serve, arrange 5 agnolotti on each serving plate. Top with radicchio, walnuts and sage. Pour over the browned butter and top with some freshly ground black pepper.

CARLA'S TIP If you're having trouble sourcing radicchio, use whatever bitter greens are currently in season as they're great for aiding digestion.

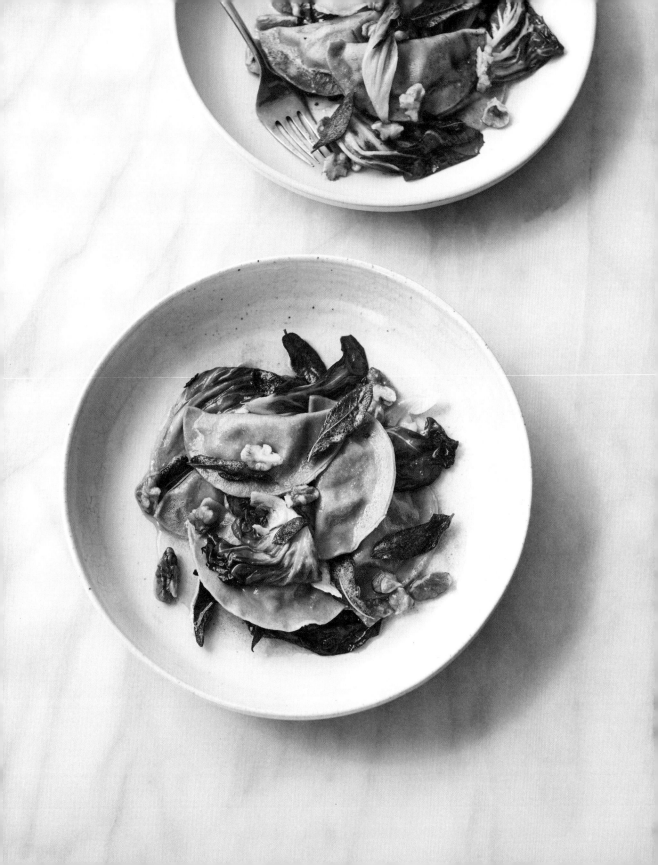

Tangy Tempeh Green Curry

Making curry paste is super easy, and it ensures you avoid the hidden additives and preservatives contained in packaged alternatives. With ginger acting as a powerful anti-inflammatory alongside basil (which may inhibit an enzyme that causes inflammation in the body), this paste is perfect for the healing phase of the program.

SERVES 4

3 teaspoons extra-virgin coconut oil or ghee
300 g (10½ oz) tempeh, cut into bite-sized pieces
200 g (7 oz/1 medium) green capsicum (bell pepper), cut into thin strips
240 g (8½ oz, about 2 small) zucchini (courgettes), diced
200 g (7 oz) Japanese pumpkin (squash), diced
250 ml (8½ fl oz/1 cup) tinned coconut milk
250 ml (8½ fl oz/1 cup) Vegetarian Broth (page 229), or water
125 ml (4 fl oz/½ cup) water
120 g (4½ oz) green beans, trimmed
1½ tablespoons freshly squeezed lime juice, or to taste
1 large handful coriander (cilantro) stems & leaves, coarsely chopped, plus extra for garnish
sea salt & freshly ground black pepper, to taste

Curry Paste
1 teaspoon ground coriander
1 teaspoon ground cumin
2 green chillies, seeds removed, finely chopped
2 tablespoons fresh ginger, finely chopped
1 large handful coriander (cilantro), coarsely chopped
1 large handful basil, chopped
zest of ½ unwaxed lime
1 tablespoon extra-virgin coconut oil

To prepare the curry paste, combine all ingredients in a high-speed blender and blend until smooth.

Heat 2 teaspoons of the coconut oil in a large saucepan over a medium heat. Cook the tempeh for 2 minutes on each side until slightly golden. Remove and set aside.

Melt the remaining coconut oil in the pan over a medium heat. Add the curry paste and stir for 30 seconds, or until fragrant. Add the capsicum, zucchini, pumpkin, coconut milk, broth and water and stir to combine. Bring to the boil, then reduce to a simmer and cook for 10 minutes, or until the vegetables are just tender and the liquid is reduced by a third.

Add the cooked tempeh and green beans and gently simmer for 2–3 minutes, or until the beans are just cooked through. Add the lime juice and stir through the fresh coriander. Season the dish with salt and pepper and garnish with the additional coriander to serve.

CARLA'S TIP This curry is definitely mild, so if you like a little spice add some fresh red chilli to the curry paste.

Gluten Free   Dairy Free   Vegetarian   Vegan   Stage 1 Friendly   Low FODMAP

Vegetable, Tapenade & Béchamel Bake

This recipe channels the '80s, but I still love devouring a good veggie bake, especially when it involves layers of savoury olive and creamy béchamel. This is a gutsy recipe, literally, with so many fibre-filled ingredients to help your beneficial bugs work hard at making short-chain fatty acids, which are anti-inflammatory, immune boosting and good for your metabolic health and wellbeing.

SERVES 4

400 g (14 oz, about 2 medium) red capsicum
(bell pepper)
300 g (10½ oz, about 1 medium) sweet potato, peeled
& cut lengthways into 1.5 cm (½ in) thick slices
extra-virgin olive oil, for cooking
240 g (8½ oz, about 2 small) zucchini (courgettes),
trimmed & cut lengthways into 1 cm (½ in) thick
slices
300 g (10½ oz, about 1 medium) eggplant (aubergine),
trimmed & cut lengthways into 1 cm
(½ in) thick slices

Béchamel Sauce
2 tablespoons cultured butter or extra-virgin olive oil
30 g (1 oz/¼ cup) arrowroot
625 ml (21 fl oz/1½ cups) almond milk, heated
3 tablespoons nutritional yeast flakes,
plus extra for sprinkling
sea salt, to taste

Tapenade
75 g (2¾ oz/½ cup) pitted kalamata olives
3 handfuls flat-leaf (Italian) parsley leaves

Preheat the oven to 200°C (400°F/Gas Mark 6).

Place the capsicum on an oven tray. Roast for 35–40 minutes until the skin is blistered and the flesh has softened. Put in a bowl, cover and set aside to cool, then peel and de-seed.

Place the sweet potato on an oven tray. Drizzle with oil and roast for 20–25 minutes until just tender.

Place the zucchini on an oven tray. Drizzle with oil and roast for 15–20 minutes until just tender.

Preheat a large frying pan over a medium–high heat. Drizzle the eggplant with oil and cook for 1–2 minutes on each side until browned and tender. Transfer to a plate and set aside.

Decrease the oven temperature to 180°C (350°F/Gas Mark 4).

For the béchamel sauce, melt the butter in a medium saucepan over a low–medium heat. Add the arrowroot. Cook for 1 minute, stirring with a wooden spoon until it begins to foam. Switch to a whisk and gradually pour in the milk, whisking continuously until well incorporated to prevent lumps. Add the yeast flakes. Continue to whisk, increase the heat to medium and cook for 3–5 minutes until thick enough to coat the back of a spoon. Season with salt. Cover with a piece of baking paper and set aside.

To prepare the tapenade, blend the olives and parsley in a small food processor until finely chopped. Alternatively, finely chop by hand and mix in a small bowl. Set aside.

To assemble, put a layer of sweet potato in the base of a 20 × 20 cm (8 × 8 in) square baking tray or ovenproof dish. Pour over a thin layer of béchamel, add a layer of zucchini, then the tapenade. Next, add a layer of capsicum, another thin layer of béchamel, then finish with a layer of eggplant and cover with the remaining béchamel. Sprinkle with yeast flakes.

Cover with foil and bake for 30 minutes, then uncover and bake for a further 10 minutes, or until the surface is golden. Slice to serve.

Cauliflower & Tempeh Falafel with Tahini Sauce

These balls of yumminess are as moreish as they are versatile. A great dinner, lunch or afternoon snack, they are sure to become a household favourite! Tempeh is a wonderful plant-based source of protein, and one of the few soy products that can actually be beneficial for your gut. It's also a very good source of manganese, fibre and copper, all essential for good digestive health.

SERVES 4 (Makes 20 falafel balls)

30 g (1 oz/¼ cup) arrowroot
1 free-range organic egg, lightly beaten
150 g (5½ oz/1 cup) white sesame seeds, for coating
coconut oil, for shallow frying
Broccoli & Asparagus Tabouleh (page 200), to serve

Cauliflower & Tempeh Falafel
400 g (14 oz) cauliflower, stalk & florets,
    coarsely chopped
300 g (10½ oz) packet tempeh, coarsely chopped
1 garlic clove
2 teaspoons ground cumin
1 teaspoon sea salt
1 teaspoon ground coriander
¼ teaspoon cayenne pepper

Tahini Sauce
60 ml (2 fl oz/¼ cup) tahini
2 tablespoons water
1½ tablespoons freshly squeezed lemon juice
1½ tablespoons extra-virgin olive oil
sea salt, to taste

To prepare the falafel, blend all ingredients in a food processor until finely chopped.

Put the arrowroot, egg and sesame seeds in separate bowls. Using your hands, compact and roll the falafel mixture into 20 golf ball–sized balls. Roll in arrowroot to lightly coat, shaking off any excess. Dip in egg and roll in sesame seeds to coat. Arrange on a tray and refrigerate for 20 minutes.

Meanwhile, prepare the tahini sauce by whisking all ingredients in a small bowl. Set aside.

Pour coconut oil into a medium frying pan to a depth of 2 cm (¾ in). Place over a medium heat. The oil is at the right temperature when a small piece of falafel dropped in floats straight to the surface, bubbling and gently browning. Cook the falafel in batches, turning frequently, for 6–8 minutes until golden on all sides. Transfer onto some paper towel to drain.

You can also cook your falafel in the oven: arrange on a tray, drizzle with coconut oil and bake at 200°C (400°F/Gas Mark 6) for 45 minutes, turning occasionally, until browned all over.

Serve with Broccoli & Asparagus Tabouleh and the tahini sauce.

CARLA'S TIP For a vegan-friendly version, simply swap the egg for tinned coconut milk during the coating process.

Gluten Free   Dairy Free   Vegetarian   Vegan Option   Stage 3 Friendly

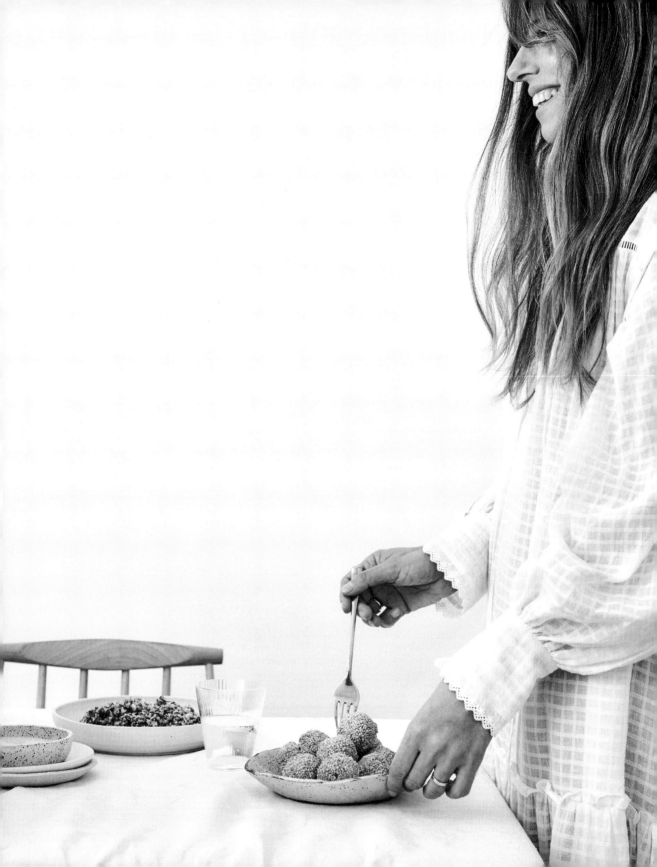

Spring Tart with Asparagus, Peas & Herbs

Tarts always look impressive, but they are really so easy to create – a wonderful one-dish meal that is as delicious for dinner as it is for breakfast or lunch the next day. Buckwheat flour and almond meal ensure this pastry is gluten free, while inulin hero asparagus is music to our microbiome. As inulin is a non-digestible prebiotic, it passes through our digestive system unabsorbed, fermenting and fuelling the beneficial bacteria, and fighting off inflammation-causing parasites, harmful bacteria and yeast.

SERVES 6

115 g (4 oz) salted cultured butter, diced & chilled, plus
    extra for greasing
150 g (5½ oz/1 cup) buckwheat flour
100 g (3½ oz/1 cup) ground almonds
30 g (1 oz/¼ cup) arrowroot
1½ tablespoons water, chilled
1 tablespoon unpasteurised apple-cider vinegar

Filling

320 g (11½ oz/2 bunches) asparagus, woody ends
    trimmed, cut in half crossways
70 g (2½ oz/½ cup) frozen peas, thawed
2 spring onions (scallions), white part only,
    thinly sliced
1 small handful mint, coarsely chopped
1 small handful basil, coarsely chopped
1 small handful flat-leaf (Italian) parsley leaves,
    coarsely chopped
100 g (3½ oz) goat's feta, crumbled
6 free-range organic eggs
160 ml (5½ fl oz/⅔ cup) almond milk
sea salt & freshly ground black pepper

CARLA'S TIP If you don't tolerate goat's feta well, simply omit it and sprinkle nutritional yeast through the filling for a nice cheesy flavour.

LOW-FODMAP OPTION Swap the asparagus and green peas for zucchini (courgette) and capsicum (bell pepper), ensuring you don't exceed the low-FODMAP quantities. Zucchini is low FODMAP at 65 g (2¼ oz) per serve, green capsicum at 52 g (1¾ oz) per serve. There is no limit on red capsicum. Use the green part of the spring onion instead of the white.

Recipe continues >

Gluten Free　　　Vegetarian　　　Stage 4 Friendly　　　Low-FODMAP Option

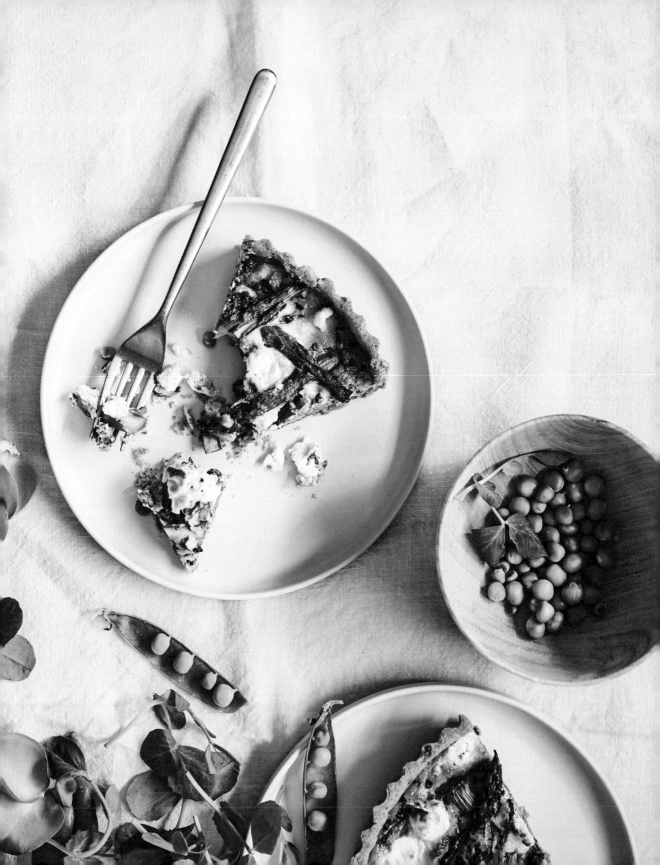

Preheat the oven to 180°C (350°F/Gas Mark 4). Lightly grease a 25 cm (10 in) round, 3 cm (1¼ in) deep, loose-based fluted tart tin with cultured butter. Refrigerate to chill.

To prepare the pastry, blend the buckwheat flour, ground almonds and arrowroot in a food processor. Add the butter and blend until the mixture resembles coarse crumbs. Add the water and vinegar, then blend until the mixture begins to bind. Turn it out onto a clean kitchen bench and shape into a disc. Wrap in plastic wrap and refrigerate for 30 minutes.

Roll out the dough between two sheets of baking paper so that it is slightly larger than the prepared tin and approximately 5 mm (¼ in) thick. Carefully lay it over the tin and press down to cover the base and sides. Trim around the edge and use any leftover scraps to patch up cracks. Prick the base with a fork several times. Cover with a piece of baking paper and fill the tin with baking weights, uncooked rice or dry beans. Bake the tart shell for 10 minutes, then remove the baking weights and paper and bake for a further 5 minutes, or until crisp and golden brown. Remove from the oven and set aside to cool slightly.

Toss the asparagus, peas, spring onion and herbs in a medium bowl. Pile the filling into the tart shell and top with the feta.

Lightly beat the eggs and milk in a medium bowl. Season with salt and pepper and pour over the vegetables and cheese.

Bake the tart for 30–35 minutes until the egg is set and the top is golden brown. Leave in the tin for 10 minutes to cool slightly, then remove and slice to serve. This tart can be served warm, at room temperature or chilled.

Lentil Moussaka

I crave moussaka every so often, and I find that it never fails to satisfy. It is hearty, flavoursome and generous in its offering of layered goodness. This vegetarian version of moussaka is made with fibre-rich lentils, along with fragrant and flavoursome spices such as cinnamon, which help soothe digestive discomfort and may inhibit the growth of certain pathogenic bacteria. Paired with a healthy version of 'béchamel', this lovely recipe tastes even better the next day.

SERVES 4–6

extra-virgin olive or coconut oil, for cooking
900 g–1 kg (2 lb–2 lb 3 oz, about 3 medium) eggplants
    (aubergine), cut lengthways into 1 cm (½ in) thick
    slices

Lentil Sauce
220 g (8 oz/1 cup) dried puy lentils, thoroughly rinsed
splash of unpasteurised apple-cider vinegar
2 tablespoons extra-virgin coconut oil
1 medium onion, finely chopped
1 medium leek, white part only,
    halved lengthways & thinly sliced
2 garlic cloves, finely chopped
1½ teaspoons ground cinnamon
¾ teaspoon ground nutmeg
½ teaspoon ground allspice
2 × 400 g (14 oz) tinned tomatoes
500 ml (17 fl oz/2 cups) water
1 large strip kombu, rinsed
sea salt & freshly ground black pepper, to taste

Béchamel
1 litre (34 fl oz/4 cups) almond milk
    or other nut-based milk
½ medium onion, finely diced
1 bay leaf
6 parsley stalks, finely diced
80 g (2¾ oz) cultured salted butter
60 g (2 oz/½ cup) arrowroot
½ teaspoon sea salt
½ teaspoon ground nutmeg, plus extra for sprinkling

CARLA'S TIP Make two trays of this moussaka and
store one in the freezer for a last-minute dinner option.

Recipe continues >

Pre-soak the lentils in a large bowl full of warm water with a splash of apple-cider vinegar for at least 7 hours (or overnight). Drain, rinse and change the water and vinegar 1–2 times over the soaking period. Drain and set aside.

To prepare the lentil sauce, heat the oil in a medium saucepan over a low–medium heat. Cook the onion, leek and garlic until softened. Add the spices and cook for 30 seconds, or until fragrant. Add the tomatoes and stir to combine. Add the water, pre-soaked lentils and kombu and bring to the boil. Cover the saucepan and reduce to a simmer. Cook for 45 minutes, or until the lentils are tender and the sauce is thick. Remove and discard the kombu. Season with salt and pepper.

Meanwhile, preheat a large frying pan over a medium–high heat. Brush the eggplant with oil on both sides. Grill in batches for 2–3 minutes on each side until browned. Transfer to a tray and set aside until required.

To prepare the béchamel, heat the milk, onion, bay leaf and parsley stalks in a medium saucepan and bring to a simmer. Remove from the heat and set aside for 10 minutes to infuse.

Strain the milk, discarding the onion, bay leaf and parsley stalks. In a separate medium saucepan, melt the butter over a low–medium heat. Add the arrowroot and, stirring with a wooden spoon, cook for 2 minutes, or until it becomes foamy. Gradually pour in the hot milk, whisking continuously, until incorporated to make a smooth sauce. Simmer over a low heat, whisking occasionally, for 5–10 minutes to thicken. Add the salt and nutmeg and whisk to combine.

Preheat the oven to 180°C (350°F/Gas Mark 4).

To assemble the moussaka, arrange half of the grilled eggplant to cover the bottom of a square, 25 cm × 5 cm (10 in × 2 in) deep baking dish. Spread half the lentil mixture on top, followed by half the béchamel. Repeat these layers. Sprinkle the top with some nutmeg and bake for 30 minutes, or until the sauce begins to bubble up the sides.

Leave to cool for a few minutes before slicing the moussaka to serve. Moussaka can be prepared and cooked up to 3 days in advance. Bring back to room temperature before reheating.

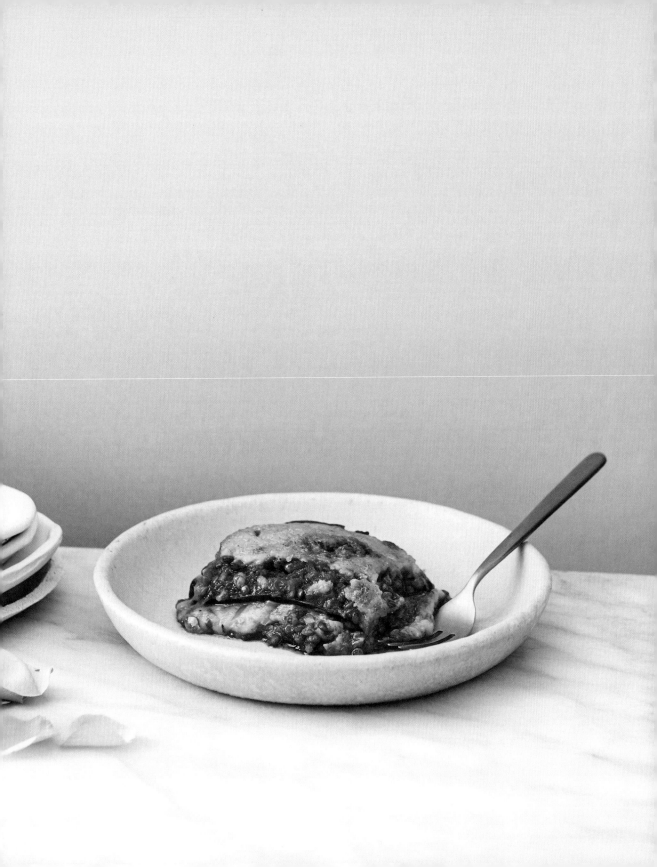

Spiced Carrot & Tempeh Fritters

Tempeh is a fermented soy product that boasts a lovely nutty flavour and can be used in stir-fries, curries, stews and fritters. It is not only rich in bone-boosting calcium, digestive enzyme–promoting manganese and anti-inflammatory isoflavones, but it also happens to be gut-friendly, making it a great plant-based protein. Thanks to the fermentation process, which helps break down the phytic acid in soybeans, tempeh is easier to digest and full of postbiotics.

MAKES 12

2 teaspoons coriander seeds
1½ teaspoons cumin seeds
400 g (14 oz) carrot, peeled & coarsely grated
300 g (10½ oz) tempeh, coarsely grated
1 large handful coriander (cilantro) stems & leaves,
    coarsely chopped
1 teaspoon sea salt
½ teaspoon freshly ground black pepper
3 free-range organic eggs, lightly beaten
ghee or extra-virgin olive oil, for cooking
wilted spinach dressed with extra-virgin olive oil &
    lemon juice, to serve

Lemon Coconut Yoghurt
180 g (6½ oz/¾ cup) coconut yoghurt
1½ tablespoons freshly squeezed lemon juice

In a small frying pan, lightly toast the coriander and cumin seeds over a low–medium heat for 30 seconds, or until fragrant. Coarsely grind using a mortar and pestle or a spice grinder.

Put the spices in a medium bowl with the carrot, tempeh, coriander, salt and pepper and mix well to combine. Stir through the lightly beaten eggs.

In a large frying pan, melt 1–2 teaspoons of ghee over a medium heat. Drop small mounds of batter (about ¼ cup) into the pan and flatten using the back of a spatula until the fritters are approximately 8 cm (3¼ in) in diameter. Cook for 3–4 minutes on each side until golden brown and cooked through. Transfer the fritters to a plate and place in the oven on low to keep warm.

To make the lemon coconut yoghurt, whisk the ingredients in a small bowl. Dollop some over the fritters and serve with wilted spinach.

LOW-FODMAP NOTE This recipe is low FODMAP at three fritters per serve.

Ginger & Miso Sweet Potato Soup with Wakame

When you combine prebiotic ingredients such as wakame with probiotic ingredients such as miso, you get what is referred to in the science world as a 'synbiotic', where two compounds are working in synergy to support healthy bacteria in the gut. This warming, slightly sweet, slightly umami soup also contains a host of antioxidant-rich, anti-inflammatory vegetables – the perfect cleanse and reset.

SERVES 4

1½ tablespoons dried instant wakame flakes

1 tablespoon coconut oil, extra-virgin olive oil or ghee

1 medium onion, diced

1 medium carrot, peeled & diced

1 celery stalk, diced

500 g (1 lb 2 oz) sweet potato, peeled & diced

1 tablespoon fresh ginger, finely grated

1 litre (34 fl oz/4 cups) Vegetarian Broth or chicken Bone Broth (page 229), or store-bought stock

90 g (3 oz/⅓ cup) shiro (white) miso paste

2 tablespoons freshly squeezed lemon juice

Soak the wakame in cold water for 10 minutes, or until rehydrated. Drain and set aside.

Heat the oil in a medium saucepan over a low heat. Sauté the onion, carrot and celery until softened, about 3–4 minutes. Add the sweet potato and ginger and stir to combine. Pour in the broth, bring to the boil, then reduce to a gentle simmer. Cover and cook for 20 minutes, or until the sweet potato is tender.

Add the miso and lemon juice and stir to combine. Remove the soup from the heat to cool slightly and, using an electric or hand-held blender, blend until smooth. Return to the heat to warm through, but do not boil.

Serve the soup topped with the rehydrated wakame.

CARLA'S TIP If you're making this with the vegetarian version of Bone Broth (page 229), reduce the amount of miso added to the soup. I'd start with 1 tablespoon and do a taste test – it's the best way to know how much extra to add.

LOW-FODMAP OPTION Reduce the wakame to 1 tablespoon. Use the green part of a leek instead of the onion, reduce the sweet potato to 300 g (10½ oz) and supplement with 200 g (7 oz) white potato such as Nicola or Carisma. You will also need to reduce the amount of miso to 45 g (1½ oz).

Gluten Free   Dairy Free   Vegetarian   Vegan   Stage 3 Friendly   Low-FODMAP Option

Okra, Roasted Tomato & Buckwheat Noodle Bowl with Miso Ginger Broth

This lovely recipe is one of my all-time favourite soups. It features okra, also known as 'lady's fingers'. Mild in flavour, with a textural, sticky quality, this highly nutritious vegetable is a great source of fibre and antioxidants, including anti-inflammatory and anti-histamine quercetin. It has been used in traditional Asian medicine to help protect against inflammatory gastric diseases. I really enjoy this soup with tofu, but I only eat it very occasionally, as I believe unfermented soy is best consumed in moderation.

SERVES 4

250 g (9 oz) cherry tomatoes, halved

250 g (9 oz) 100% buckwheat noodles

2 tablespoons dried instant wakame flakes

1 litre (34 fl oz/4 cups) Vegetarian Broth or chicken Bone Broth (page 229), or store-bought stock

250 ml (8½ fl oz/1 cup) water

2 tablespoons ginger, peeled & very thinly sliced

250 g (9 oz) soft (not silken) tofu, cut into bite-sized pieces

200 g (7 oz) okra, halved lengthways

60 g (2 oz/¼ cup) shiro (white) miso paste

1 tablespoon tamari

1 teaspoon black sesame seeds, toasted

1 teaspoon white sesame seeds, toasted

togarashi, for sprinkling, to serve

Preheat the oven to 200°C (400°F/Gas Mark 6).

Arrange the tomatoes cut-side down on a small baking tray. Roast for 10 minutes, or until the skins begin to blister and the tomatoes are soft, but are still holding their shape. Set aside.

Bring a medium saucepan of water to the boil. Cook the buckwheat noodles, referring to packet instructions until al dente. Drain, cool and set aside.

Soak the wakame in cold water for 10 minutes, or until rehydrated. Drain and set aside.

To prepare the miso ginger broth, combine the broth, water and ginger in a medium saucepan over a medium heat and bring to the boil. Decrease the heat and simmer for 5 minutes. Add the tofu and okra and simmer for 2–3 minutes until the okra is just tender but still has a slight bite.

In a small bowl, blend the miso and tamari with approximately 125 ml (4 fl oz/½ cup) of the broth. Pour the mix into the miso ginger broth, gently stirring to combine.

To serve, divide the noodles between deep serving bowls. Top with the okra, tofu, roasted tomato and wakame. Pour over the ginger broth and sprinkle with sesame seeds and togarashi.

CARLA'S TIP If you're not vegetarian, make sure to make the miso ginger broth with chicken bone broth – it will help to soothe and seal the gut. You can also swap the tofu for some steamed chicken or fish; simply slice or flake it and add to serve.

LOW-FODMAP OPTION Reduce the amount of miso to 45 g (1½ oz).

Gluten Free   Dairy Free   Vegetarian   Vegan   Stage 2 Friendly   Low-FODMAP Option

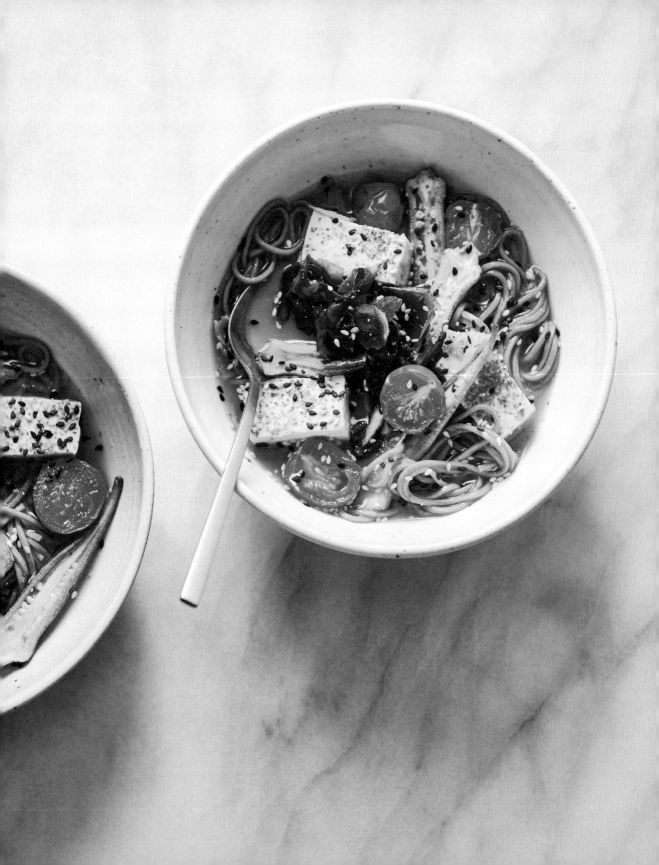

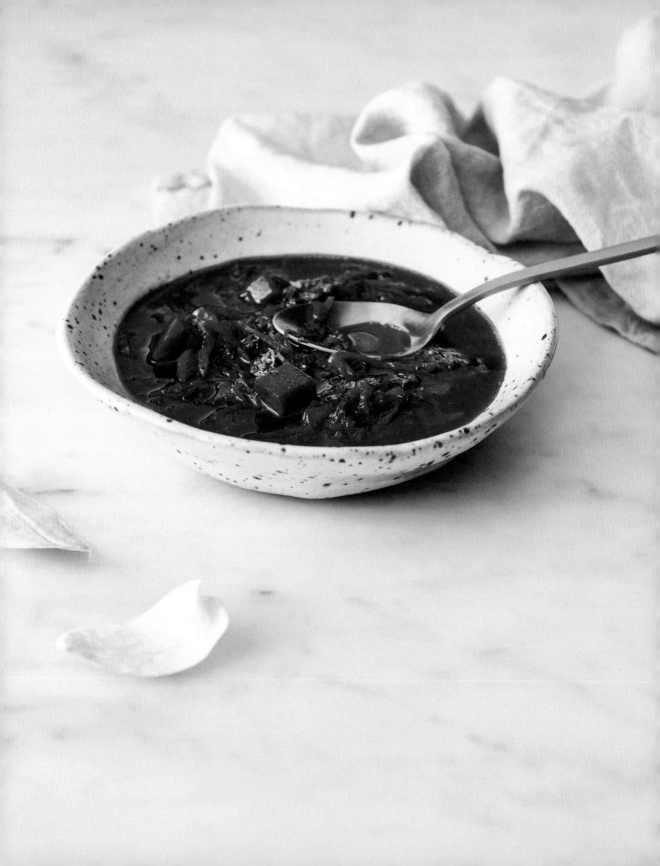

Beet & Daikon Soup
with Rocket Pesto

An old Chinese proverb says that 'eating pungent radish and drinking hot tea let the starved doctors beg on their knees'. Daikon, or Chinese radish, is actually a cruciferous vegetable, detoxifying as well as anti-inflammatory and excellent for boosting digestive function. The beautiful red pigment in beetroot, which is also a great liver detoxifier, comes from betalain, an antioxidant and anti-inflammatory. Betalain is being explored for its long-term effects on inflammation, with short-term studies showing impressive anti-inflammatory benefits.

SERVES 4

500 g (1 lb 2 oz/about 2 large) beetroot (beets)

2 teaspoons caraway seeds

2 tablespoons extra-virgin olive oil

1 medium onion, finely sliced

2 garlic cloves, finely chopped

120 g (4½ oz/½ cup) carrot, coarsely grated

480 g (1 lb 1 oz/2 cups) daikon (white radish), coarsely grated

400 g (14 oz) red cabbage, finely shredded

1.5 litres (51 fl oz/6 cups) Vegetarian Broth or beef Bone Broth (page 229), or store-bought stock

60 ml (2 fl oz/¼ cup) unpasteurised apple-cider vinegar

sea salt & freshly ground black pepper, to taste

coconut yoghurt or kefir, to serve (optional)

Rocket Pesto

80 g (2¾ oz) rocket (arugula) leaves

125 ml (4 fl oz/½ cup) extra-virgin olive oil

To keep from staining your hands as you work with the beetroot, wear gloves. Coarsely grate one beetroot and cut the other into 1 cm (½ in) cubes.

Toast the caraway seeds in a medium frying pan over a low heat for 30 seconds, or until fragrant. Set aside in a small bowl.

Using the same pan, heat the oil over a low heat. Sauté the onion and garlic until softened, about 1 minute. Add the beetroot, carrot, daikon, cabbage and toasted caraway seeds and stir to combine. Pour in the broth and bring to the boil. Reduce the heat to low and cook at a gentle simmer for 25–30 minutes, or until the beetroot is tender.

Meanwhile, blend the rocket and oil for the pesto in a small food processor until finely chopped. Transfer to a small bowl and set aside.

Add the vinegar to the soup and stir to combine. Season with salt and pepper.

Serve topped with a generous dollop of rocket pesto and yoghurt, if desired.

CARLA'S TIP Meat eaters can substitute beef Bone Broth for Vegetarian Broth for added gut benefits.

Gluten Free   Dairy Free   Vegetarian   Vegan   Stage 2 Friendly

Roasted Jerusalem Artichoke Soup

If you are looking for a soup with an incredible depth of flavour, as well as getting to the guts of it (literally), this is it. The evidence is mounting around the benefits of Jerusalem artichokes on gut health. Why? Inulin. Acting as a prebiotic, inulin has the ability to stimulate the growth of beneficial bacteria. I love roasting the artichokes before blending them with the other ingredients – it really brings out a nutty depth and goes perfectly with sautéed leek.

SERVES 4

1 kg (2 lb 3 oz) Jerusalem artichokes, scrubbed
60 ml (2 fl oz/¼ cup) ghee, coconut or extra-virgin olive oil, melted to room temperature
1 medium onion, coarsely chopped
½ medium leek, white part only, thickly sliced
1 celery stalk, coarsely chopped
2 garlic cloves, coarsely chopped
5 thyme sprigs
1.25 litres (42 fl oz/5 cups) Vegetarian Broth or chicken Bone Broth (page 229), or store-bought stock
180 ml (6 fl oz/¾ cup) almond milk
60 ml (2 fl oz/¼ cup) freshly squeezed lemon juice
sea salt & freshly ground white pepper, to taste
extra-virgin olive oil, for drizzling

Preheat the oven to 200°C (400°F/Gas Mark 6).

Arrange the artichokes on a roasting tray. Add 1 tablespoon of the ghee and toss to coat evenly. Roast the artichokes for 45 minutes, or until golden brown and tender.

Melt the remaining ghee in a medium saucepan over a low–medium heat. Sauté the onion, leek, celery and garlic for 4–5 minutes, or until softened. Add the roasted artichokes, thyme, broth and almond milk and bring to the boil. Reduce to a simmer and cook for 10–15 minutes, or until the vegetables are tender.

Remove from the heat and discard the thyme sprigs. Using a hand-held blender, blitz the soup until smooth. Add the lemon juice, season with salt and pepper and serve drizzled with some olive oil.

CARLA'S TIP Jerusalem artichokes are a strong prebiotic, and for some people they can cause loud tummy rumbles and discomfort – especially if there is still a gut imbalance. So consume with care, especially if your digestive system is very sensitive.

Gluten Free   Dairy-Free Option   Vegetarian   Vegan Option   Stage 3 Friendly

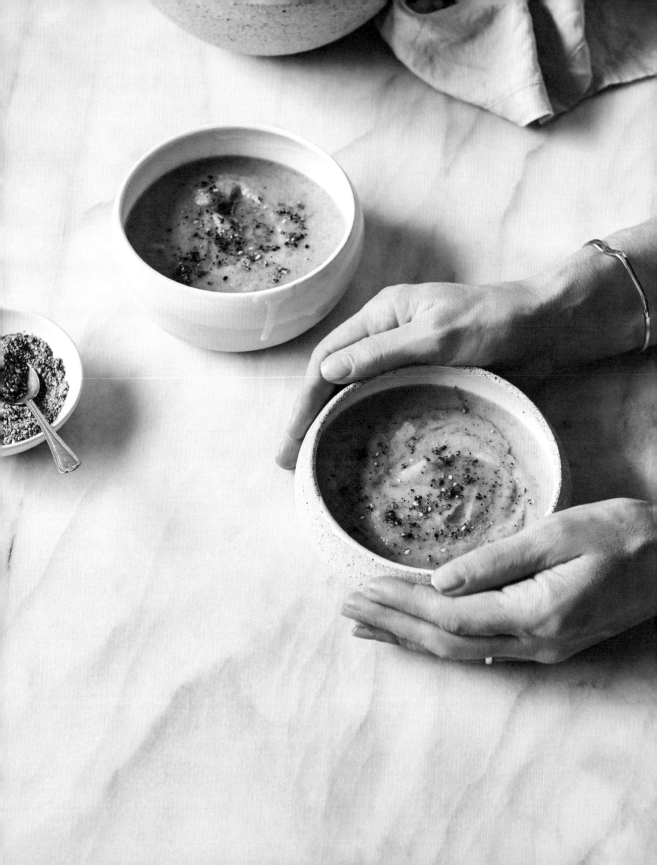

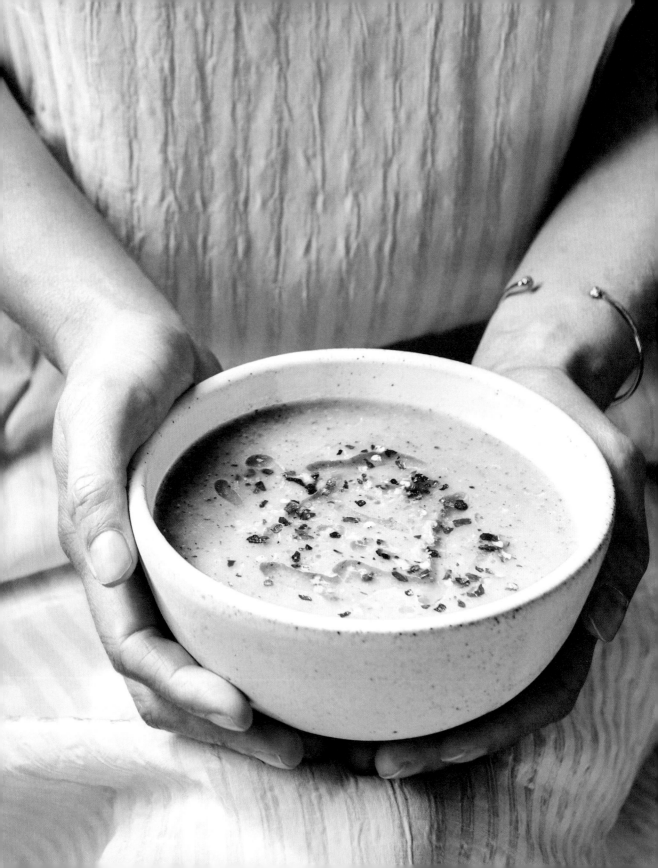

Zucchini, Fennel, Mint & Basil Soup

This flavoursome anti-inflammatory soup is a quick and easy one-pot dish full of nourishing vegetables and broth. Fennel boasts calming and anti-spasmodic properties and is wonderful for digestive health. And the herbs aren't just there to brighten the dish – basil contains powerful plant compounds including eugenol, citronellol and linalool that have been shown to help reduce gut inflammation.

SERVES 4

2 tablespoons extra-virgin olive oil

1 small or medium fennel bulb, trimmed, thickly sliced, fronds reserved

1 medium onion, finely sliced

1 garlic clove, finely chopped

450 g (1 lb, about 3 medium) zucchini (courgettes), thickly sliced

2 handfuls basil

2 handfuls mint

1 litre (34 fl oz/4 cups) Vegetarian Broth or chicken Bone Broth (page 229), or store-bought stock

1½ tablespoons freshly squeezed lemon juice, plus zest to serve

sea salt & freshly ground black pepper, to taste

extra-virgin olive oil, to serve

dried chilli flakes, to serve

Heat the oil in a medium saucepan over a medium heat. Cook the fennel, onion and garlic until softened, about 3 minutes. Add the zucchini, basil, mint and reserved fennel fronds and stir to combine. Pour in the broth and bring to the boil over a medium heat. Reduce to a gentle simmer. Cook for 5 minutes, or until the vegetables are tender.

Add the lemon juice and season with salt and pepper. Using a high-speed or hand-held blender, blend the soup until smooth.

Serve topped with a drizzle of extra-virgin olive oil, a sprinkle of lemon zest and some chilli flakes.

CARLA'S TIP   From Stage 4, add a sprinkling of one of the Sesame Salts (page 239) for a boost in flavour and antioxidants.

Gluten Free   Dairy Free   Vegetarian   Vegan   Stage 2 Friendly

Fennel & Chive Noodle Soup

If you are feeling a little under the weather, this is the perfect dish to curl up on the couch with. Anti-inflammatory fennel helps promote digestion as well as being the perfect tummy soother. Chives are a great alternative to onion and garlic if you're eating low FODMAP, and they add a wonderful depth of flavour.

SERVES 4

2 tablespoons extra-virgin olive, plus extra for drizzling

240 g (8½ oz/2 medium) carrots, cut into 1 cm (½ in) dice

190 g (6½ oz/1 small) fennel bulb, trimmed & thinly sliced, fronds reserved

1 litre (34 fl oz/4 cups) Vegetarian Broth or chicken Bone Broth (page 229), or store-bought stock

240 g (8½ oz, about 2 small) zucchini (courgettes), diced

100 g (3½ oz) 100% buckwheat noodles, broken into quarters to form short pieces & cooked according to packet instructions

1 bunch chives, finely chopped

sea salt & freshly ground black pepper, to taste

Heat the oil in a medium saucepan over a medium heat. Cook the carrot and fennel until beginning to soften, about 3 minutes. Pour in the broth and bring to the boil. Reduce to a gentle simmer, add the zucchini and cook for 3 minutes, or until the vegetables are tender.

Add the buckwheat noodles, chives and fennel fronds and cook for 1 minute, or until the noodles are heated through. Season with salt and pepper to taste and serve topped with a drizzle of olive oil.

CARLA'S TIP If you have any leftover roasted chicken in the refrigerator, shred and add it to your soup for a hit of protein. Or if you'd like to keep it veggie-friendly, poach an egg and add it on top for a sort of egg drop soup.

Gluten Free   Dairy Free   Vegetarian   Vegan   Stage 1 Friendly   Low FODMAP

Parsnip, Leek & Apple Soup
with Walnut Dukkah

I enjoy being inventive with my vegetable soups, combining flavoursome ingredients – spices, herbs, seeds, nuts and sometimes, fruit. Parsnips provide a subtle, earthy sweetness, highlighted by the sourness and slight acidity of green apple, and, together with the leeks, help stimulate the growth of beneficial bacteria.

SERVES 4

2 tablespoons ghee, extra-virgin olive or coconut oil

2 leeks, white part only, sliced into rounds

4 medium parsnips, coarsely chopped

1 large green apple, peeled & cored

1 tablespoon thyme

1 bay leaf, fresh or dried

1 litre (34 fl oz/4 cups) Vegetarian Broth or chicken
 Bone Broth (page 229), or store-bought stock

125 ml (4 fl oz/½ cup) coconut cream

sea salt & freshly ground black pepper

extra-virgin olive oil, to serve

Walnut Dukkah

1 tablespoon coriander seeds

2 teaspoons cumin seeds

1 teaspoon fennel seeds

60 g (2 oz/½ cup) walnuts, finely chopped

35 g (1¼ oz/¼ cup) white sesame seeds

sea salt & freshly ground black pepper

Heat the ghee in a large saucepan over a low–medium heat. Cook the leek for 10 minutes, or until softened. Add the parsnips, apple, thyme and bay leaf and stir to combine. Pour in the broth and bring to the boil over a high heat. Decrease the heat and simmer for 20 minutes, or until the parsnip softens.

Meanwhile, to make the walnut dukkah, toast the coriander, cumin and fennel seeds in a small frying pan over a low heat for 30 seconds, or until fragrant. Coarsely grind using a spice grinder or pestle and mortar.

Return the small frying pan to the heat and lightly toast the walnuts and sesame seeds until golden brown. Add the spice mix and toss to combine. Season with salt and pepper and transfer to a small bowl.

Remove the soup from the heat and discard the bay leaf. Add the coconut cream and, using a high-speed or hand-held blender, blend the soup until smooth. Season with some salt and pepper, return to the heat and warm through.

Serve each bowl of soup with a generous drizzle of olive oil and a sprinkling of walnut dukkah.

CARLA'S TIP Walnuts are rich in skin and gut-loving omega-3s. Studies show that this superfood helps increase the diversity of our microbiome by stimulating the growth of several bacteria, including *Lactobacillus*.

LOW-FODMAP OPTION Swap the white part of the leek for the green part and the apple for a large carrot; it'll add a beautiful colour and a little natural sweetness!

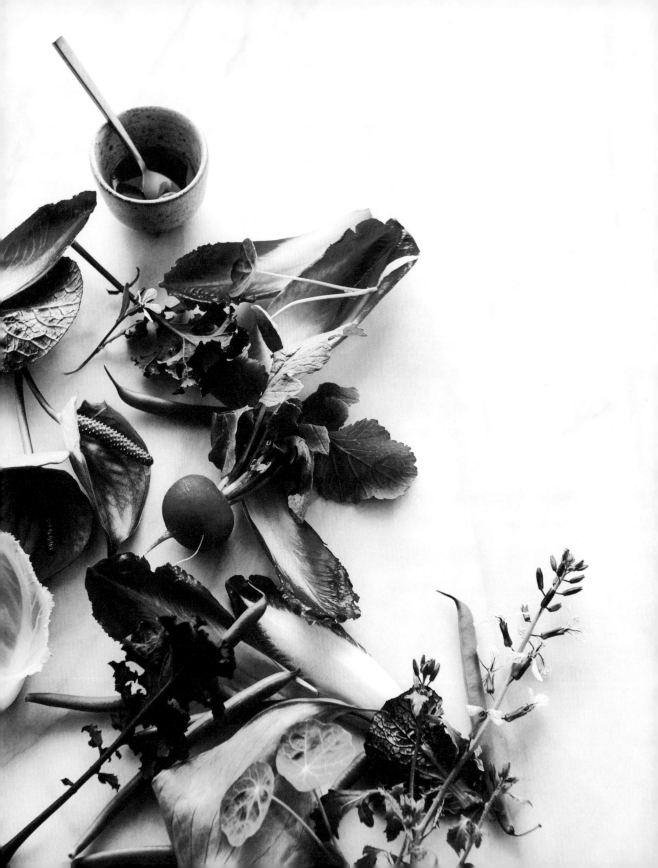

Sides & Snacks

Sweet Potato Chips with Lime Cream

Sweet potato chips are moreish, and the lime cream in this recipe takes them to another level of deliciousness. While I try to stay mostly dairy free when on a gut cleanse, a small amount of goat's or sheep's yoghurt gives lots of nourishment without the tummy compromise. This is because goat's and sheep's milk have smaller fat globules than cow's milk, and a higher proportion of medium-chain fatty acids, making them easier to digest. While coriander offers anti-fungal properties, you can swap it for rosemary if you like, to give this recipe an Italian twist and to reap some added anti-inflammatory benefits.

SERVES 4

2 tablespoons arrowroot

1 teaspoon sea salt

900 g (2 lb, 2 large) sweet potatoes, skin left on, scrubbed & cut into 1 cm (½ in) thick 'chips'

extra-virgin coconut oil, warmed, for drizzling

30 g (1 oz/⅓ cup) flaked almonds, lightly toasted

¼ teaspoon dried chilli flakes

1 large handful coriander (cilantro) stems & leaves, coarsely chopped

Lime Cream

180 g (6½ oz/¾ cup) sheep's, goat's or coconut yoghurt

1 tablespoon extra-virgin olive oil

zest of 1 unwaxed lime

1 tablespoon freshly squeezed lemon juice

sea salt, to taste

Preheat the oven to 200°C (400°F/Gas Mark 6) and line two large baking trays with baking paper.

In a large bowl, combine the arrowroot and salt. Add the sweet potato chips in batches and toss to coat. Shake off any excess and arrange the chips in a single layer across the two trays. Drizzle with coconut oil and bake for 20–25 minutes, turning once, until tender, crisp and golden.

Meanwhile, prepare the lime cream by whisking all ingredients in a small bowl.

Serve the sweet potato chips scattered with flaked almonds, chilli flakes and coriander, with the lime cream on the side.

LOW-FODMAP OPTION Swap the sweet potato for carrots. Cook for an extra 10 minutes, or until tender. Reduce the sheep's or goat's yoghurt to 125 g (4½ oz/½ cup) or swap for coconut yoghurt. Carrots are a good source of the prebiotic arabinogalactan, shown to increase the production of short-chain fatty acids that help the body fight inflammation.

Gluten Free   Dairy-Free Option   Vegetarian   Vegan Option   Stage 3 Friendly   Low-FODMAP Option

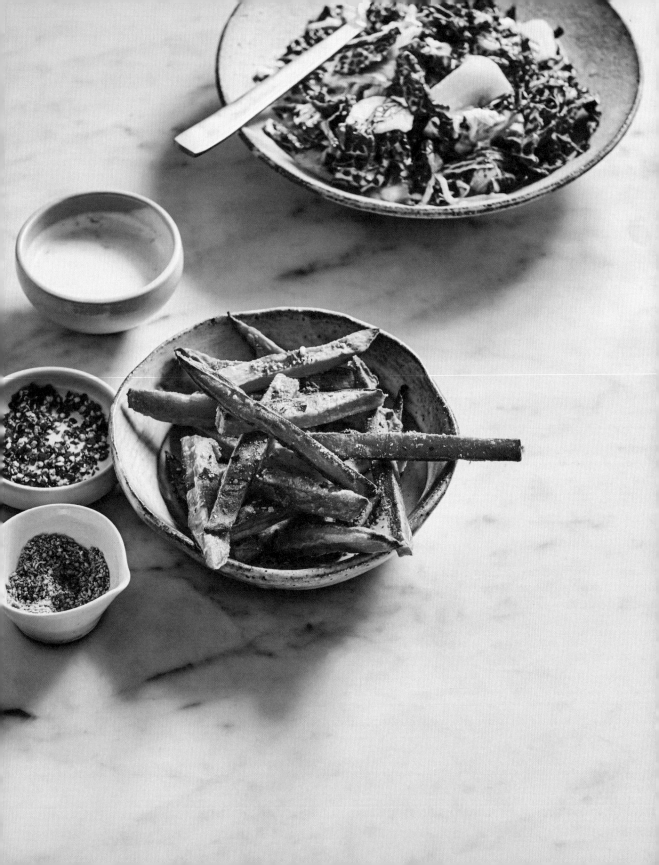

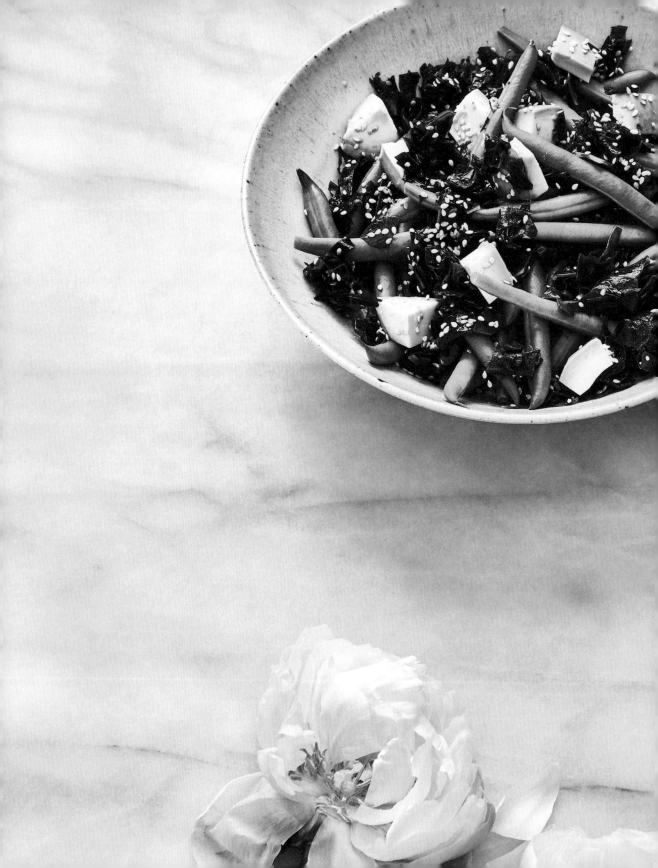

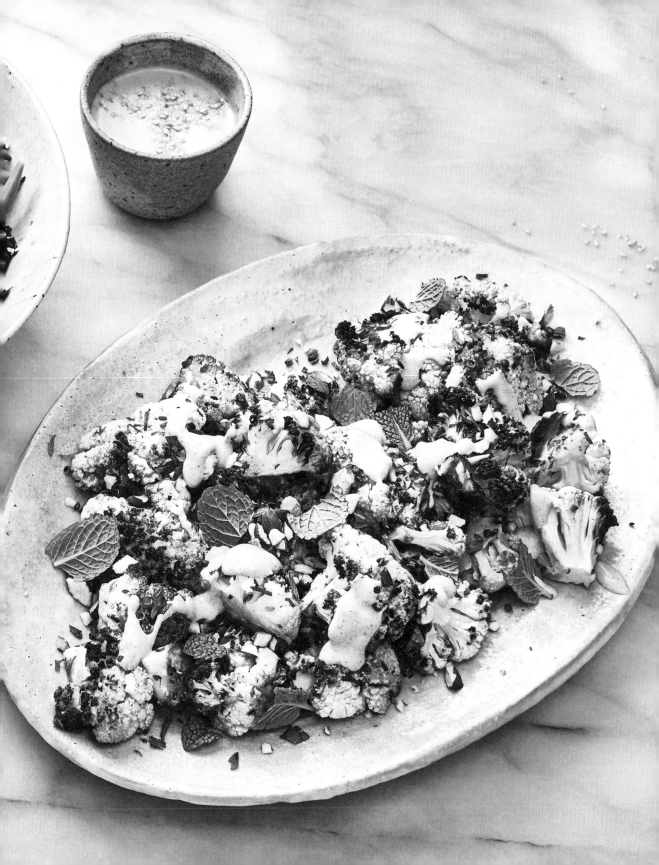

Creamed Cruciferous

Gluten Free   Dairy-Free Option
Vegetarian   Vegan Option
Stage 4 Friendly

*What's the secret to a healthy gut microbiota?
Cruciferous vegetables. If you are not a fan of these
'aromatic' greens, then put them in this lovely,
creamy sauce and you may feel very differently.
Silverbeet, kale and cabbage all contain distinct
compounds shown to promote microbial diversity.
Adding onion and garlic to the mix gives a boost
of prebiotic inulin to feed the beneficial bugs,
while nutritional yeast flakes are a flavoursome
and dairy-free alternative to parmesan cheese.*

SERVES 2

1 tablespoon ghee or extra-virgin olive oil
½ medium onion, sliced
1 garlic clove, finely chopped
1 bunch silverbeet (Swiss chard), stems only,
     thinly sliced
200 ml (7 fl oz) tinned coconut milk
3 tablespoons nutritional yeast flakes
175 g (6 oz) kale leaves (minus their stems),
     coarsely chopped
250 g (9 oz) Chinese cabbage (wombok),
     coarsely chopped
sea salt & freshly ground black pepper, to taste

Heat the ghee in a large frying pan over a low–
medium heat. Add the onion, garlic and silverbeet
stems and cook until softened, about 2 minutes.
Pour in the coconut milk and bring to the boil
over a medium heat. Reduce to a simmer and
add the yeast flakes. Cook for 2–3 minutes, or until
the sauce is slightly thickened. Add the kale and
cabbage, stirring occasionally, until wilted. Season
with salt and pepper to serve.

Green Beans with Miso, Tahini & Umeboshi Dressing

Gluten Free   Dairy Free
Vegetarian
Stage 2 Friendly

*Pairing miso and tahini dressing with some steamed
green beans topped with sesame seeds with a simple
piece of fish is a beautiful option for a healthy dinner
that entices and satisfies. We love green beans for
their high fibre and phytonutrient content, but also
for their levels of silica, which helps strengthen
connective tissue and reduce inflammation of the
digestive tract.*

SERVES 4–6

10 g (¼ oz/½ cup) dried instant wakame flakes
300 g (10½ oz) green beans, trimmed,
     blanched & cooled
1 avocado, cut into 2 cm (¾ in) chunks
2 tablespoons white sesame seeds, toasted
80 ml (2½ fl oz/⅓ cup) Miso, Tahini & Umeboshi
     Dressing (page 245)

Soak the wakame in cold water for 10 minutes,
or until rehydrated. Drain and set aside.

In a medium bowl, combine the wakame,
blanched beans, avocado and sesame seeds.
Add the dressing and toss to combine.
Leftover dressing can be stored in an airtight
container for up to 1 week.

Image page 192

CARLA'S TIP Feel free to use whatever vegetables
are in season: zucchini (courgette), broccoli and
sugarsnap peas would be great in this dish too.

Spice-Roasted Cauliflower with Nut Butter Cream, Almonds & Herbs

Image page 193

If you know anyone who is sitting on the fence about cauliflower, this is the dish that may convert them. The spices bring a Middle Eastern flair, and the nut butter cream gives it a lovely rich texture, but they also each bring a host of anti-inflammatory, antispasmodic and digestion-boosting properties.

SERVES 4–6

600 g (1 lb 5 oz) cauliflower, cut into florets
2 teaspoons coriander seeds
2 teaspoons cumin seeds
1 teaspoon caraway seeds
60 ml (2 fl oz/¼ cup) ghee or extra-virgin olive oil
80 g (2¾ oz/½ cup) activated almonds, coarsely chopped
1 large handful flat-leaf (Italian) parsley leaves, coarsely chopped
1 large handful mint, coarsely chopped
45 g (1½ oz/⅓ cup) pomegranate seeds (optional)

Nut Butter Cream
100 ml (3½ fl oz) coconut cream
80 g (2¾ oz/⅓ cup) almond butter
80 ml (2½ fl oz/⅓ cup) freshly squeezed lemon juice
2 teaspoons ground cumin
1 teaspoon ground coriander
½ teaspoon sea salt

Preheat the oven to 220°C (430°F/Gas Mark 7) and arrange the cauliflower florets across two large baking trays.

In a small frying pan, lightly toast the coriander, cumin and caraway seeds over a low heat for 30 seconds, or until fragrant. Coarsely grind the spices using a mortar and pestle or spice grinder, then return to the pan. Add the ghee and heat until melted, then drizzle the mix over the cauliflower. Bake for 30 minutes, or until the florets are tender and the tips are golden.

Meanwhile, prepare the nut butter cream by blending all ingredients in a small food processor until smooth.

To serve, drizzle the roasted cauliflower with some nut butter cream and scatter with almonds, parsley, mint and pomegranate, if desired.

Sides & Snacks

CARLA'S TIP Pomegranates are a great source of fibre as well as anti-inflammatory antioxidants. Studies show that they may also help stimulate the production of *Lactobacilli*.

Gluten Free   Dairy-Free Option   Vegetarian   Vegan Option   Stage 3 Friendly   195

Roasted Carrot, Witlof & Toasted Walnut Salad with Orange & Umeboshi Dressing

I love the bitterness of witlof paired with the sweetness of baby carrots and orange, dressed with tart umeboshi – what a flavoursome combo. Both carrots and witlof (similar to radicchio in flavour) are a very good source of pro-vitamin A, which is vital for supporting healthy mucous membranes in the gut and skin. Witlof is also a good source of fibre and helps promote the secretion of bile, which aids the liver and gall bladder in digestion. This superfood also contains a potent flavonoid called kaempferol, which pre-clinical studies show possesses antioxidant, antimicrobial, anti-inflammatory and anti-cancer properties.

SERVES 4

135 g (5 oz/¾ cup) black or tri-colour quinoa, thoroughly rinsed

375 ml (12½ fl oz/1½ cups) water

500 g (1 lb 2 oz, approx. 1 bunch) Dutch carrots, tops trimmed

2 tablespoons ghee or olive oil

1 teaspoon ground coriander

200 g (7 oz, approx. 2-3 heads) witlof, leaves separated

1 large handful mint

35 g (1¼ oz /⅓ cup) walnuts, toasted & coarsely chopped

Dressing
finely grated zest of 1 unwaxed orange

60 ml (2 fl oz/¼ cup) freshly squeezed orange juice

2 umeboshi salted plums, pitted

2 tablespoons extra-virgin olive oil

1 tablespoon warm water

2 teaspoons manuka honey

freshly ground black pepper, to taste

CARLA'S TIP If witlof is unavailable, substitute radicchio or other bitter salad leaves such as rocket (arugula) or chicory (endive). Goat's cheese can make a flavoursome addition, and according to Monash University it is low FODMAP at 40 g (1½ oz) per serve.

Preheat the oven to 200°C (400°F/Gas Mark 6).

In a medium saucepan, combine the quinoa and water and bring to the boil. Cover and reduce the heat to a gentle simmer. Cook the quinoa for 15 minutes until almost all of the water has been absorbed. Remove the pan from the heat and let sit, covered, for another 5 minutes, or until the quinoa's 'tails' have sprouted and the remaining water has been absorbed.

Spread the quinoa out on a tray and set aside to cool. Arrange the carrots in a baking tray, dot with ghee and sprinkle with ground coriander. Roast for 15 minutes, or until just tender and beginning to caramelise. Set aside to cool.

To make the dressing, blend all ingredients except for the pepper in a small food processor. Season with pepper.

Combine the quinoa, carrots, witlof, mint and walnuts in a large bowl. Drizzle with dressing and toss to combine.

LOW-FODMAP OPTION Use some pure organic maple syrup to sweeten the dressing.

Gluten Free   Dairy-Free Option   Vegetarian   Vegan Option   Stage 4 Friendly   Low-FODMAP Option

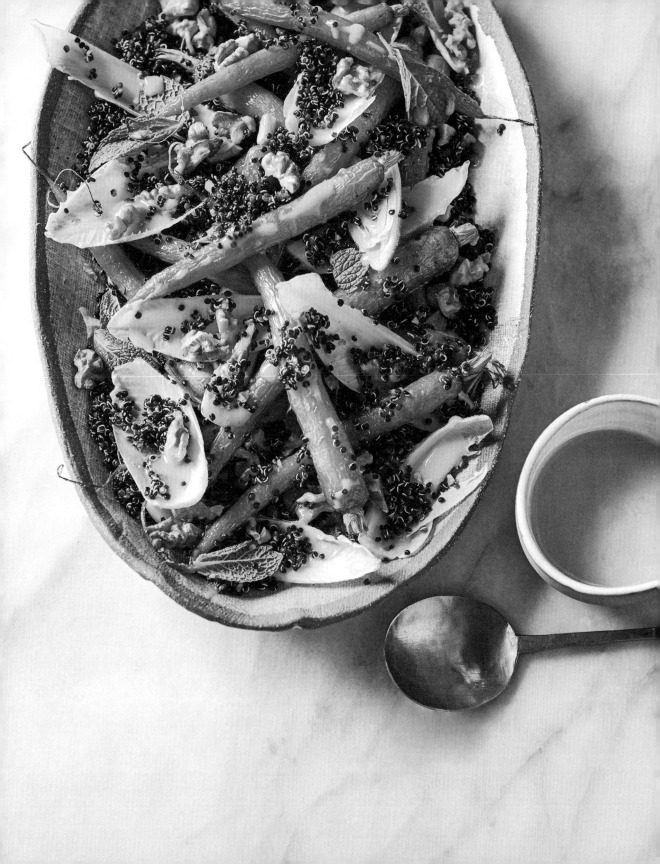

Gut-Healing Turmeric & Parsley Tabouleh

This is a fragrant, delicious and gutsy tabouleh. High in flavonoids such as quercetin, parsley helps heal the gut lining and increase bile production. Paired with anti-inflammatory and digestive enzyme–boosting turmeric and lemon, this recipe is great on its own or paired with our Spiced Chicken, Three Ways (page 144) or Pick-Your-Own-Herbs Oven-Baked Barramundi (page 134).

SERVES 2

90 g (3 oz/½ cup) quinoa, rinsed thoroughly
325 ml (11 fl oz/1⅓ cups) water
1 teaspoon ground turmeric
2 handfuls flat-leaf (Italian) parsley leaves,
    finely chopped
1 handful mint, finely chopped
zest of 1 unwaxed lemon
1½ tablespoons freshly squeezed lemon juice
1 tablespoon extra-virgin olive oil
sea salt & freshly ground black pepper, to taste

In a medium saucepan, combine the quinoa and water and bring to the boil. Cover and reduce the heat to a gentle simmer. Cook for for 15 minutes until almost all of the water has been absorbed. Remove the pan from the heat and let sit, covered, for another 5 minutes, or until the quinoa's 'tails' have sprouted and the remaining water has been absorbed. Stir through the turmeric.

Spread the quinoa out on a tray and set aside to cool. In a medium bowl, combine the parsley and mint and stir. Add the cooled quinoa and stir it through the herbs. Dress the quinoa with the lemon zest, juice and olive oil and toss to combine. Season with salt and freshly ground black pepper.

CARLA'S TIP Swap the quinoa for cooked buckwheat for another Stage 1–friendly version of this delicious tabouleh. If you are not partial to quinoa, white basmati rice can be substituted from Stage 2 onwards. Diced tomato and cucumber can be added for extra fibre from Stage 3.

Gluten Free   Dairy Free   Vegetarian   Vegan   Stage 1 Friendly   Low FODMAP

Green Beans, Sautéed Fennel, Capers & Herbs

When I was little, the green beans that accompanied our meals were often a very unappetising brownish-green colour. This recipe celebrates the vibrant greenness of beans and the detoxifying chlorophyll that makes them that beautiful, intense hue. An array of fragrant, digestive-strengthening herbs brightens this dish, and capers always add a spark of intense flavour – and quercetin, which helps tighten the junctions between the cells of the gut wall.

SERVES 4

300 g (10½ oz) green beans, trimmed

1½ tablespoons extra-virgin olive oil or ghee

190 g (6½ oz, 1 small) fennel bulb, trimmed
& thinly sliced

2 tablespoons capers, drained, rinsed
& coarsely chopped

zest of 1 unwaxed lemon

1½ tablespoons freshly squeezed lemon juice

1 large handful dill, coarsely chopped

1 large handful mint, finely chopped

1 large handful flat-leaf (Italian) parsley leaves,
finely chopped

1 tablespoon extra-virgin olive oil

freshly ground black pepper, to serve

Bring a medium saucepan full of water to the boil. Blanch the beans for 30 seconds until just tender but still firm to the bite. Drain and refresh in a bowl of ice water.

Heat the ghee in a large frying pan over a medium heat. Cook the fennel, tossing occasionally, for 3–4 minutes until just tender. Add the beans, capers and lemon zest, toss to combine, and allow the beans to cook for long enough to warm through.

Add the lemon juice, herbs and oil and toss to combine. Season with pepper.

CARLA'S TIP Add some flaked salmon to this lovely salad for some protein, transforming it from a side to a main meal.

LOW-FODMAP OPTION Keep your consumption of fennel to 48 g (1¾ oz) or less per serve, and beans to 75 g (2¾ oz, about 15 beans) or less per serve.

Gluten Free   Dairy Free   Vegetarian   Vegan   Stage 1 Friendly   Low FODMAP

Broccoli & Asparagus Tabouleh

This wheat-free, nutrient-dense tabouleh is rich in ingredients that will supercharge your gut microbiota. Every ingredient has myriad gut-boosting benefits, with anti-inflammatory broccoli, inulin-rich asparagus and crunchy pumpkin seeds, which provide a good dose of zinc for gut repair.

SERVES 4

1 teaspoon sea salt, plus extra to taste

40 g (1½ oz/¼ cup) pumpkin seeds (pepitas)

35 g (1¼ oz/¼ cup) sunflower kernels

300 g (10½ oz/approx. 1 medium head) broccoli, broken into florets & stem coarsely chopped

160 g (5½ oz/1 bunch) asparagus, woody ends trimmed & cut into halves

2 handfuls flat-leaf (Italian) parsley leaves, finely chopped

1 large handful mint, finely chopped

1 small handful oregano

2 spring onions (scallions), white part only, finely chopped

zest & juice of 1 unwaxed lemon

2 tablespoons extra-virgin olive oil

1 garlic clove, finely chopped

Fill a medium bowl three-quarters of the way with warm water. Add the salt and stir until mostly dissolved. Add the pumpkin seeds and sunflower kernels, cover the bowl with a clean tea towel (dish towel) and set aside in a warm place to soak for at least 7 (and up to 12) hours. Drain and rinse.

Blanch the broccoli and asparagus in boiling water for 3–5 minutes, or until just tender while retaining a bit of crunch. Refresh in a bowl of iced water and drain.

Pulse the cooled broccoli and asparagus in a food processor until finely chopped. Transfer to a medium bowl and add the parsley, mint, oregano and spring onion. Stir to combine.

Pulse the drained sunflower kernels and pumpkin seeds in the food processor until finely chopped. Add to the greens with the lemon zest and juice, olive oil and garlic. Toss to combine.

CARLA'S TIP I love to add the bitter green chicory (endive) to this tabouleh as it is not only delicious, but adds to the digestive enzyme–boosting properties of this lovely recipe.

Gluten Free   Dairy Free   Vegetarian   Vegan   Stage 3 Friendly

Miso, Potato & Eggplant Salad

White potatoes are high GI, which is why I only eat them occasionally. However, the great news is that when you cool them, their GI lowers and they become higher in resistant starch, which our beneficial microbes love. This salad is so delicious and creamy, with an unexpected twist that works. We know miso and eggplant are like peas in a pod, but marrying them with potato is a taste revelation. Eggplant is great for your gut too, high in antioxidants and fibre to help keep your tummy protected and you regular.

SERVES 4

750 g (1 lb 11 oz, approx. 4 medium) Nicola or Carisma potatoes, peeled & cut into 3 cm (1¼ in) cubes
60 ml (2 fl oz/¼ cup) extra-virgin coconut oil
500 g (1 lb 2 oz, approx. 1 large) eggplant (aubergine), very thinly sliced into rounds
2 spring onions (scallions), white part only, thinly sliced into rounds
45 g (1½ oz/⅓ cup) pomegranate seeds (optional)

Creamy Miso Dressing
125 g (4½ oz/½ cup) red miso paste
60 ml (2 fl oz/¼ cup) warm water
2 tablespoons freshly squeezed lemon juice
2 tablespoons extra-virgin olive oil

In a medium saucepan, cover the potato with cold water and bring to the boil. Simmer for 10 minutes, or until just tender when pierced with a skewer or knife. Strain and set aside to cool completely.

Heat 1 tablespoon of the coconut oil in a large frying pan over a medium–high heat. Cook the eggplant in batches, for 30–60 seconds on each side, until tender and browned in spots. Add more oil between batches if required. Transfer the cooked eggplant to a plate and set aside.

To make the dressing, whisk all ingredients in a small bowl.

Put the cold potato, spring onions, eggplant, pomegranate seeds, if using, and miso dressing in a medium bowl and toss to combine.

CARLA'S TIP Those with irritable bowel syndrome should be aware that this double dose of nightshades (potato and eggplant) may make symptoms worse.

Gluten Free   Dairy Free   Vegetarian   Vegan   Stage 4 Friendly

Baked Postbiotic Kimchi

When you cook probiotic foods, don't worry too much about heating and destroying the live bacteria. More and more research shows that even when heated, fermented foods contain bioactive compounds called postbiotics. These bacterial by-products may have all sorts of benefits: anti-inflammatory, immunomodulatory, anti-obesogenic, anti-hypertensive and more. They seem to be heat resistant too! This dish is not only bio-active, but delicious, rich and creamy and full of flavour – the perfect accompaniment to a piece of fish or chicken.

SERVES 4

300 g (10½ oz/½ cup) kimchi, homemade (page 230)
    or store-bought
250 ml (8½ fl oz/1 cup) tinned coconut milk
3 tablespoons nutritional yeast flakes,
    plus extra for sprinkling

Preheat the oven to 200°C (400°F/Gas Mark 6).

Arrange the kimchi in two 3.5 cm (1½ in) deep, 375 ml (12½ fl oz/1½ cups) capacity ovenproof baking dishes.

In a small saucepan, whisk the coconut milk and yeast flakes. Simmer over a low–medium heat for 2–3 minutes until reduced slightly. Pour into the dishes to almost cover the kimchi. Sprinkle over some extra yeast flakes.

Bake for 15 minutes, or until the liquid begins to bubble up around the edges.

Remove from the oven and stand for a few minutes to cool slightly before serving. One dish is meant to be shared between two people.

CARLA'S TIP As the flavours of this recipe are quite intense and rich, I love pairing it with a piece of grilled fish or roasted chicken and a simple green salad. It also pairs well with the Chicken Katsu Don (page 147).

Gluten Free   Dairy Free   Vegetarian   Vegan   Stage 3 Friendly

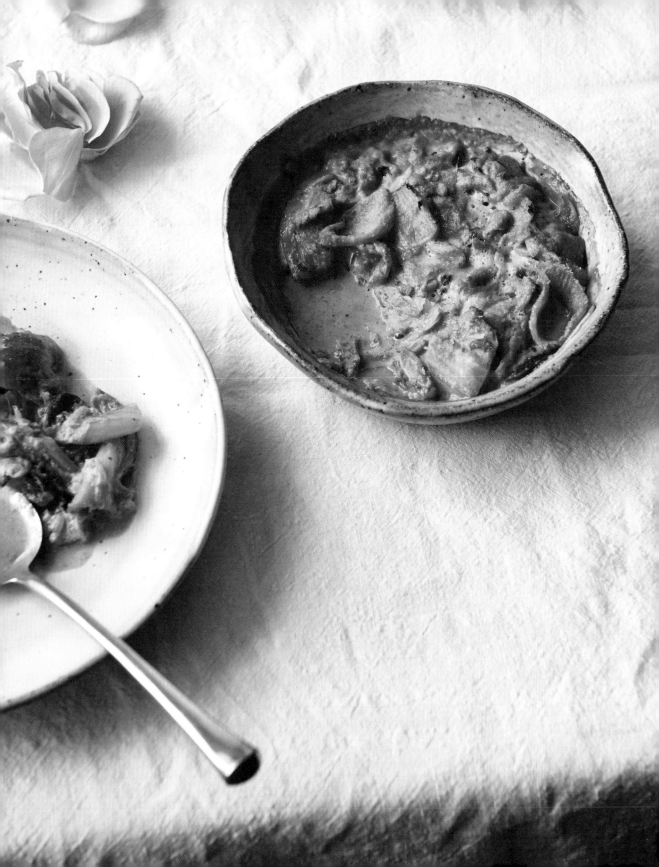

Garlicky Hummus

Image page 207

Apart from being very tasty, hummus is a great way to infuse your diet with a little extra fibre. Chickpeas contain roughly 6 to 7 g (¼ oz) of each soluble and insoluble fibre per half cup, helping to promote regularity and, subsequently, healthy digestion. I always boost my hummus with lots of garlic too. Garlic contains an indigestible fibre known as inulin, which acts as a prebiotic and promotes the growth of beneficial intestinal bacteria. I've added a beetroot version, both for its myriad health benefits and for its sweet flavour and vibrant colour.

SERVES 4–6 (Makes approx. 2 cups)

200 g (7 oz/1 cup) dried chickpeas

2 litres (68 fl oz/8 cups) warm water, plus extra for soaking

1½ teaspoons bicarbonate of soda (baking soda), plus extra for soaking

5 garlic cloves, peeled

2 tablespoons tahini, hulled or unhulled

60 ml (2 fl oz/¼ cup) freshly squeezed lemon juice

2 tablespoons extra-virgin olive oil

1 teaspoon ground cumin

sea salt & freshly ground black pepper, to taste

Beetroot-Boosted Version

250 g (9 oz/approx. 1 medium) beetroot (beet), roughly chopped (optional)

80 ml (2½ fl oz/⅓ cup) Coconut Milk Kefir (page 228)

Put the chickpeas in a medium saucepan with 1 litre (34 fl oz/4 cups) of the warm water and 1 teaspoon of the bicarb soda. Cover and set aside for 12 (and up to 24) hours. Drain, rinse and change the water and bicarb soda 1–3 times over the soaking period to prevent the chickpeas from fermenting.

Drain and rinse the chickpeas, then return to the saucepan. Cover with the remaining 1 litre (34 fl oz/4 cups) water and add the remaining bicarb soda. Bring to the boil over a high heat, then reduce to a simmer and cook for 40 minutes, or until the chickpeas are tender. Drain, reserving 60 ml (2 fl oz/¼ cup) of the cooking liquid.

Combine the chickpeas, garlic, tahini, lemon juice, olive oil and cumin in a food processor. If you're boosting your hummus with beetroot, add it now. Blend, scraping down the sides occasionally until smooth. Add a little of the cooking liquid at a time, adjusting the consistency as desired.

Season with salt and pepper. Top with coconut kefir to serve if you're making the beetroot-boosted option.

Store the hummus in an airtight container in the refrigerator for up to 1 week.

CARLA'S TIP This hummus makes a nice addition to the Pick-Your-Own-Herbs Oven-Baked Barramundi (page 134) and the Spiced Chicken, Three Ways (page 144). I also love to spread it on a piece of Prebiotic Superseed Bread (page 242) for a quick, nutritious breakfast, or on Buckwheat & Caraway Crackers (page 208) as a snack.

Gluten Free   Dairy Free   Vegetarian   Vegan   Stage 2 Friendly

Sides & Snacks

Artichoke & Green Olive Dip

Gluten Free
Vegetarian
Stage 4 Friendly

Dairy Free
Vegan
Low-FODMAP Option

If you haven't cooked much with artichokes, this dip is a great way to introduce this tasty, nutty-flavoured vegetable into your diet. Artichokes have been shown to increase beneficial bacteria in the gut and aid digestion by boosting the production of digestive bile. Here they are paired with olives, basil and oregano to create a very green, gut-boosting and tasty dip.

SERVES 4–6 (Makes 1¼ cups)

200 g (7 oz) canned artichoke hearts, drained
90 g (3 oz/½ cup) pitted green Sicilian olives
1 garlic clove, peeled & crushed
1 tablespoon extra-virgin olive oil
1 tablespoon freshly squeezed lemon juice
1 large handful basil, finely chopped
1 tablespoon oregano, finely chopped
sea salt & freshly ground black pepper, to taste

Blend the artichokes, olives and garlic in a food processor until finely chopped. Add the oil and lemon juice and blend to combine.

Transfer the mixture to a medium bowl. Add the basil and oregano and stir to combine. Season with salt and pepper to taste.

Use immediately or store in an airtight container in the refrigerator for up to 5 days.

Image page 207

CARLA'S TIP Spread this dip on Low-FODMAP Charcoal Flatbread (page 235), or if you are in Stage 2 and beyond, add 1 tablespoon of unhulled tahini for a creamy (and still dairy free) version of this delicious dip.

LOW-FODMAP OPTION Omit the garlic.

Zucchini Gremolata Dip

Gluten Free
Vegetarian
Stage 1 Friendly

Dairy Free
Vegan
Low FODMAP

This is a very versatile low-FODMAP dip, full of alkalising, detoxifying and anti-inflammatory zucchini and parsley. Zucchini and parsley are outstanding gut foods – they're great sources of fibre, minerals and vitamins, which help protect and strengthen the digestive system. Coriander seeds are an effective antimicrobial, and studies show that olive oil, rich in polyphenols and fatty acids, has a positive impact on our gut microbiome.

SERVES 6 (Makes 3 cups)

390 g (14 oz, about 2 large) zucchini (courgettes),
    roughly chopped
1 bunch flat-leaf (Italian) parsley leaves,
    finely chopped
2 teaspoons ground coriander
½ teaspoon smoked paprika
sea salt & freshly ground black pepper, to taste
juice & zest of 1 unwaxed lemon
2 tablespoons extra-virgin olive oil

Blitz all ingredients except the lemon juice and olive oil in a food processor, leaving the mixture a little chunky.

Using a mesh sieve, strain out any excess liquid. Transfer the dip to a bowl or airtight container. When ready to serve, dress with the lemon juice, oil, and salt and pepper. Store in the refrigerator for up to 1 week.

Image page 206

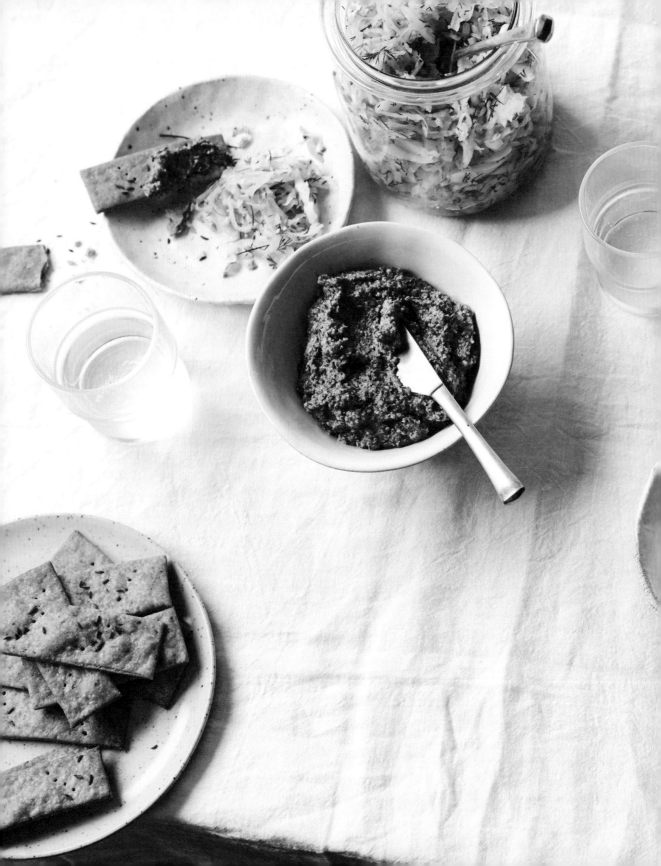

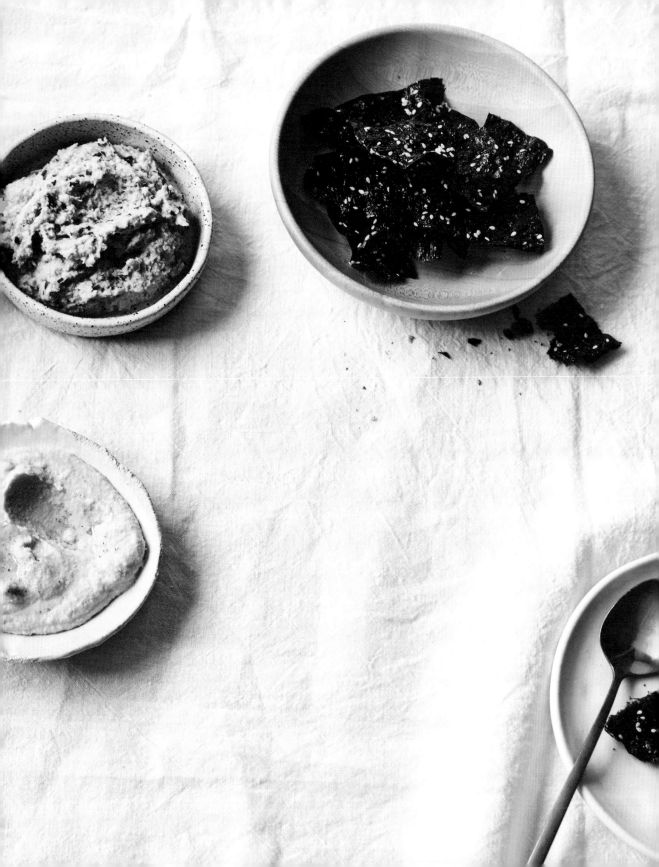

Buckwheat & Caraway Crackers

Image page 206

These are one of my all-time favourite savoury biscuits. They work just as well when entertaining (as an accompaniment to dip) as they do as a snack laden with avocado and pesto. Caraway seeds add an aromatic, earthy aniseed note. Its distinctive flavour comes from caveolins and carvones, the chemical compounds also responsible for caraway's carminative and digestive properties. Flaxseeds are packed with omega-3s and lignans – fatty acids and antioxidants that help reduce inflammation and protect the lining of the GI tract.

MAKES 32 crackers

225 g (8 oz/1½ cups) buckwheat flour
50 g (1¾ oz/½ cup) ground almonds
1 tablespoon ground golden flaxseed/linseed
1 tablespoon caraway seeds, toasted
   & coarsely ground
1 teaspoon sea salt
1 teaspoon ground cumin
60 ml (2 fl oz/¼ cup) extra-virgin olive oil
100 ml (3½ fl oz) cold water

Preheat the oven to 180°C (350°F/Gas Mark 4).

In a medium bowl, whisk the buckwheat flour, ground almonds, flaxseed, 3 teaspoons of the caraway seeds, the salt and cumin. Add the oil and cold water and stir to form a rough dough.

Turn the mixture out onto a clean kitchen bench and knead for 2 minutes, or until it forms a firm, smooth dough. Add a little extra buckwheat flour if it's sticky and a little extra water if it's dry.

Separate the dough into quarters. Work with one quarter at a time, keeping the remaining dough covered with a damp tea towel (dish towel) to prevent it drying out. Roughly shape the dough portion into a flat rectangle. Roll it out very thinly, approximately 3 mm (⅛ in) thick, between two pieces of baking paper, to make a 15 cm × 25 cm (6 in × 10 in) rectangle. Use a knife to cut eight long, rectangular crackers. Using the baking paper as a base, transfer the rectangles onto a large baking tray. Separate and space the crackers out slightly. Repeat the process with the remaining dough quarters.

Prick the crackers with the tines of a fork a few times. Brush with some water and sprinkle with the remaining caraway seeds.

Bake for 10–15 minutes, or until crisp. Remove from the oven and allow to cool.

Store the crackers in an airtight container for up to 3 weeks.

CARLA'S TIP Add 1 tablespoon of nutritional yeast flakes to the dough for a cheesy, immune-boosting cracker. Cut into larger crackers to use as a bread alternative for lunch.

Sides & Snacks

Gluten Free   Dairy Free   Vegetarian   Vegan   Stage 2 Friendly   Low FODMAP

Zucchini, Apple, Walnut & Cardamom Loaf

Just because you've given your diet a healthy overhaul doesn't mean you can't enjoy a good old-fashioned sweet loaf. This version is full of hearty goodness and is low GI, with apples and aromatic spices such as cardamom, which studies suggest may be a powerful digestive aid. Cardamom is also revered for its ability to help relieve symptoms of gastrointestinal discomfort.

SERVES 8–10

240 g (8½ oz, about 2 small) zucchini (courgettes), coarsely grated

150 g (5½ oz/1 medium) green apple, coarsely grated

120 g (4½ oz, 1 small) apple, diced

90 g (3 oz/¾ cup) walnuts, coarsely chopped

10 Medjool dates, pitted & coarsely chopped

3 free-range organic eggs, lightly beaten

60 g (2 oz/¼ cup) unsalted cultured butter, melted & cooled

1 teaspoon unpasteurised apple-cider vinegar

1 teaspoon natural vanilla extract

110 g (4 oz/¾ cup) buckwheat flour

75 g (2¾ oz/¾ cup) ground hazelnuts or almonds

30 g (1 oz/¼ cup) arrowroot

1 tablespoon chia seeds

2 teaspoons ground cardamom

1 teaspoon ground nutmeg

1 teaspoon gluten-free baking powder

½ teaspoon bicarbonate of soda (baking soda)

stevia equal to 1 tablespoon of regular sugar

Preheat the oven to 180°C (350°F/Gas Mark 4). Lightly grease and line a 20 cm × 10 cm (8 in × 4 in) loaf tin with baking paper.

In a large bowl, combine the zucchini, apples, walnuts and dates. Add the eggs, butter, apple-cider vinegar and vanilla. Stir until well combined.

In a separate bowl, whisk the buckwheat flour, ground hazelnuts, arrowroot, chia seeds, cardamom, nutmeg, baking powder, bicarb soda and stevia. Add the mix to the zucchini batter and stir to combine.

Pour into the prepared tin and bake for 50–60 minutes, or until a skewer comes out clean when inserted into the centre. Remove from the oven, cover with a clean tea towel (dish towel) and leave to cool in the tin for 10 minutes.

Turn the loaf out onto a rack to cool completely before serving.

Store in an airtight container in the refrigerator for up to 1 week. Alternatively, slice into portions and freeze in resealable bags for up to 3 months.

CARLA'S TIP This recipe makes great muffins too! Simply pour the batter into muffin tins instead of a bread tin and bake for approximately 30 minutes. Add a dollop of coconut yoghurt to serve.

Gluten Free   Vegetarian   Stage 3 Friendly

Toasted Togarashi Nori Chips

Gluten Free   Dairy Free
Vegetarian   Vegan
Stage 2 Friendly   Low FODMAP

I discovered togarashi a few years ago at a Japanese speciality store and have sprinkled it on everything from eggs and fish to sweet potato and nori chips ever since. Togarashi is a piquant seven-spice blend containing black and white sesame seeds, which boast important gut-loving nutrients such as fibre and vitamin E, while nori is a seaweed rich in gut-boosting micronutrients and inflammation-fighting antioxidants. These little chips are very addictive and are sure to become a mainstay in your cooking repertoire.

SERVES 4

10 nori sheets
2 tablespoons water
1 tablespoon tamari
2 teaspoons extra-virgin coconut oil, melted
2 teaspoons white sesame seeds
1 teaspoon togarashi

Preheat the oven to 120°C (250°F/Gas Mark 1 or 2). Line three large baking trays with baking paper.

Lay half of the nori sheets, rough side up, on a clean kitchen bench.

Combine the water, tamari and coconut oil in a small bowl. Brush the nori sheets with the mixture, going all the way around the edges. Place the remaining nori sheets on top, rough side down, pressing down to seal.

Using kitchen scissors, cut each nori square into eight strips. Arrange the strips close together on the baking trays. Brush again, then sprinkle with sesame seeds and togarashi.

Bake the chips for 15–20 minutes until dry and crisp. Set aside to cool. Serve immediately or store in an airtight container for up to 3 weeks.

Papaya with Lime Yoghurt & Toasted Coconut

Gluten Free   Dairy Free
Vegetarian   Vegan
Stage 1 Friendly   Low FODMAP

The beauty of papaya is that it is not only refreshing and cleansing to eat, but every part of it – from the seeds to the leaves and flesh – boasts impressive nutritional and medicinal properties. It also contains a powerful protein-dissolving enzyme known as papain. This makes papaya a great snack to have in-between meals as it helps our bodies break down protein and aids digestion. Coriander may seem like an outlier here, but it gives the recipe an unexpected flair and, along with the lime and coconut, has anti-microbial properties.

SERVES 2

1 small papaya
125 g (4½ oz/½ cup) coconut yoghurt
2 tablespoons freshly squeezed lime juice
2 passionfruit, halved & pulp scooped out
15 g (½ oz/¼ cup) coconut flakes, toasted
1 small handful coriander (cilantro) leaves

Cut the papaya in half lengthways. Cut off the skin, following the curve of the fruit to maintain its shape. Scoop out and discard the seeds.

Whisk the yoghurt and lime juice in a small bowl. Top the papaya with some lime yoghurt and passionfruit pulp. Scatter with coconut flakes and coriander to serve.

CARLA'S TIP Save your papaya seeds and pop them into your morning smoothie. Studies have shown that the anti-amoebic activity of these little seeds has a clearance rate ranging between 70 and 100 per cent in treating intestinal parasites. Add some macadamia nuts for Stages 3 & beyond for some added crunch and fibre.

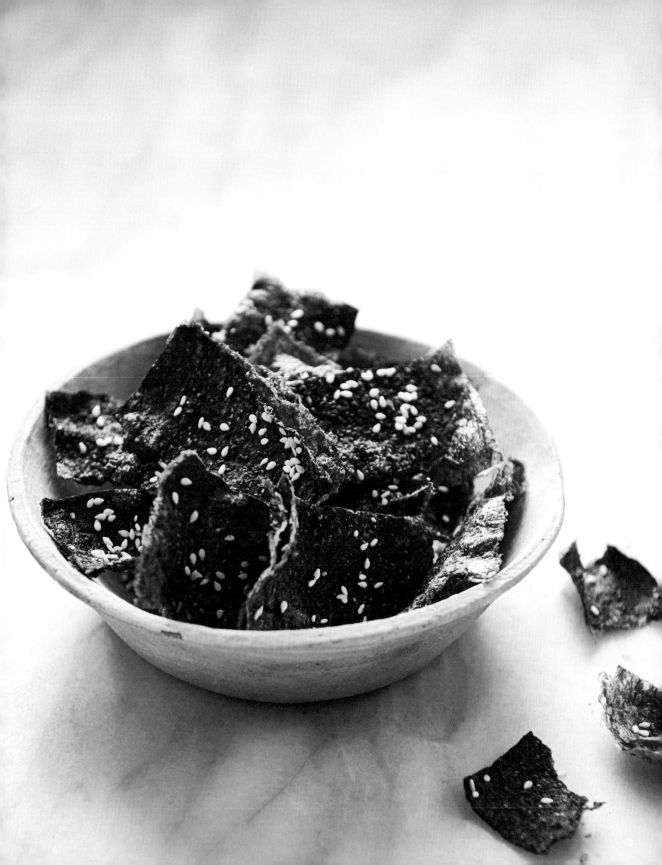

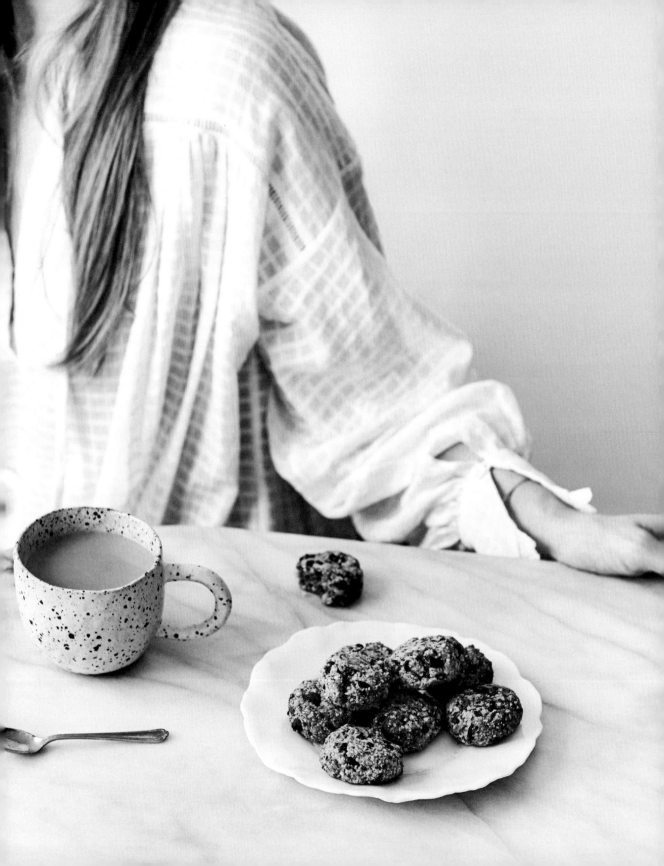

Hazelnut, Apricot & Cacao Nib Cookies

These delicious, zesty bite-sized snacks are rich in hazelnuts, which are full of vitamin E – important for helping to maintain healthy intestinal barrier function as well as healthy, skin, hair and nails. They're also a good source of monounsaturated fatty acids and fibre, promoting digestion.

MAKES 12 cookies

125 g (4½ oz/1¼ cups) ground hazelnuts
30 g (1 oz/¼ cup) arrowroot
½ teaspoon gluten-free baking powder
small pinch of sea salt
80 g (2¾ oz, about 7) organic dried sulphur-free
    apricots, finely sliced
2 tablespoons hazelnuts, coarsely chopped
2 teaspoons cacao nibs
1 free-range organic egg, lightly beaten
1½ tablespoons unsalted cultured butter, melted
2 teaspoons natural vanilla extract
finely grated zest of 1 unwaxed orange
stevia equal to 2 teaspoons regular sugar,
    or to taste

Preheat the oven to 180°C (350°F/Gas Mark 4) and line a baking tray with baking paper.

In a medium bowl, whisk the ground hazelnuts, arrowroot, baking powder and salt until combined. Add the apricots, chopped hazelnuts and cacao nibs and stir through. Add the egg, butter, vanilla and orange zest and stir until well combined. Sweeten the batter with stevia to taste.

Roll the mixture into heaped tablespoon–sized balls. Arrange on the prepared tray and flatten slightly using the back of a fork or your fingertips. The cookies will not spread as they cook.

Bake the cookies for 10–12 minutes, or until golden brown. Remove from the oven and leave on the tray for 5 minutes to cool a little. Transfer to a rack to cool completely before serving.

CARLA'S TIP I always make a double batch and pop the cookies in the freezer to have on hand if I'm craving something sweet in the afternoon. For a slightly crunchier option, flatten the cookies out a little more to a 0.5 cm (2 in) thickness.

Gluten Free   Vegetarian   Stage 4 Friendly

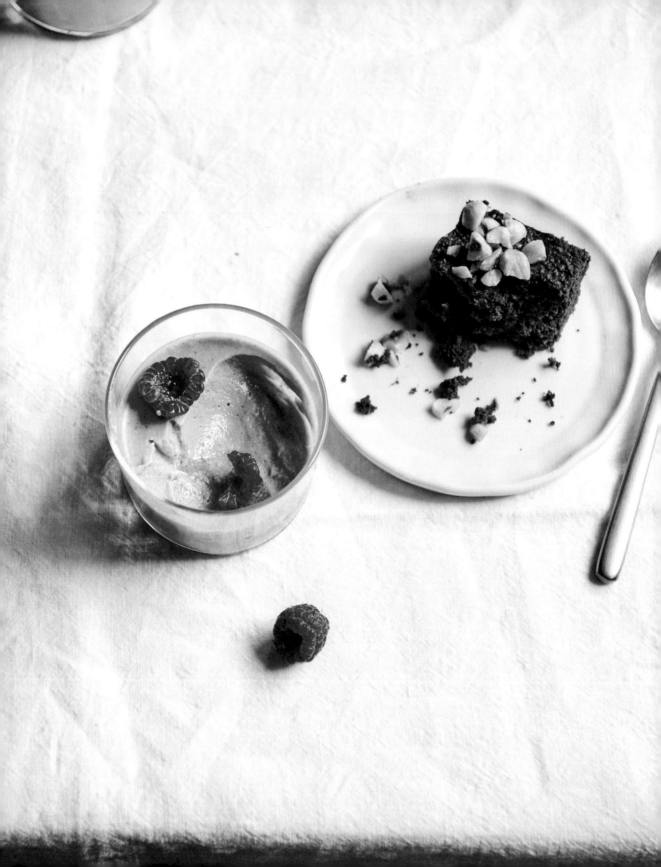

Desserts

Passionfruit Panna Cotta

Sweet, tart and creamy, this dairy-free panna cotta has all the signs of a lavish and decadent dessert, yet it is full of healthy ingredients such as lime, passionfruit, coconut and gelatin, rich in amino acids that help protect the mucosal lining of your gut.

MAKES 4

400 ml (13½ fl oz) tinned coconut milk
2 teaspoons grass-fed powdered gelatin
125 ml (4 fl oz/½ cup) passionfruit juice, strained
2 teaspoons freshly squeezed lime juice
stevia, equivalent to 1 teaspoon regular sugar,
    or to taste

Passionfruit Jelly
1 tablespoon cold water
½ teaspoon grass-fed powdered gelatin
60 ml (2 fl oz/¼ cup) passionfruit juice, strained

CARLA'S TIP This panna cotta makes a delicious snack, dessert or even breakfast paired with a little coconut yoghurt.

LOW-FODMAP OPTION Substitute tinned with unsweetened UHT coconut milk, and increase the gelatin from 2 teaspoons to 2¾ teaspoons.

To make the passionfruit jelly, pour the water into a small dish and sprinkle over the gelatin in a thin layer. Set aside for 10 minutes to bloom. Heat the passionfruit juice in a small saucepan until hot to the touch. Remove from the heat and add the gelatin, stirring to dissolve. Pour 1 tablespoon of the jelly into each base of four 125 ml (4 fl oz/½ cup) capacity moulds. Refrigerate for 30 minutes, or until just set.

To make the panna cotta, pour 80 ml (2½ fl oz/⅓ cup) of the coconut milk into a small bowl. Sprinkle over the gelatin in a thin layer and set aside for 10 minutes to bloom.

Heat the passionfruit juice in a small saucepan until hot to the touch. Remove from the heat, add the gelatin mixture and stir to dissolve. Pour in the remaining coconut milk and the lime juice and stir to combine. Sweeten with stevia to taste.

Pour the filling into the moulds over the back of a spoon (for a gentle pour and to prevent holes from forming in the jelly). Arrange on a tray and refrigerate for 4 hours, or until firm enough that the surface springs back when pressed.

To release the panna cottas from their moulds, warm the base and sides by dipping into hot water for just a few seconds. Be careful not to overheat or the panna cotta will begin to melt. Immediately invert onto serving plates. The panna cottas will hold their shape, but have a lovely wobble.

Gluten Free   Dairy Free   Stage 2 Friendly   Low-FODMAP Option

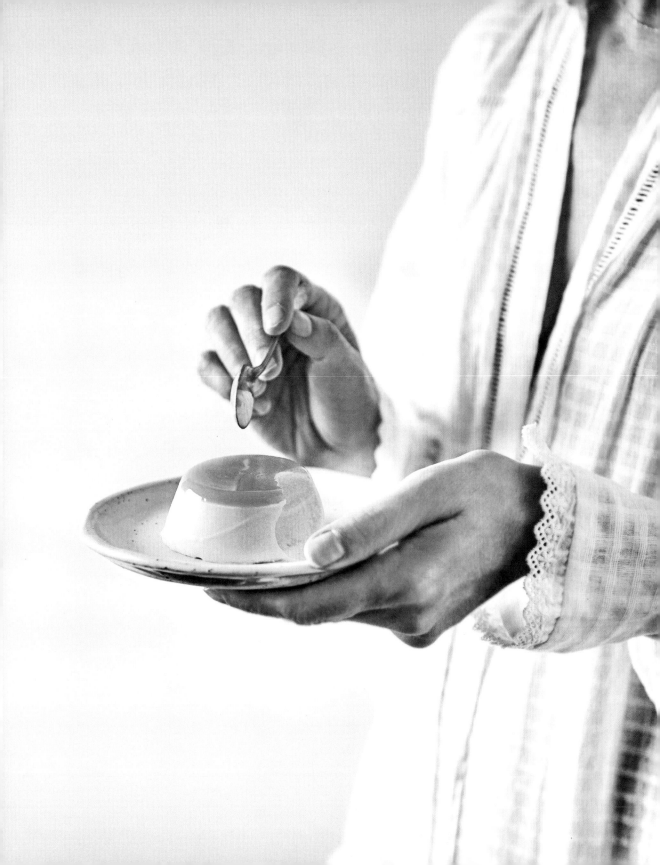

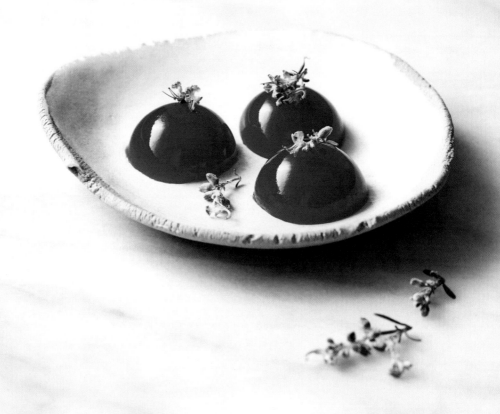

Raspberry, Licorice & Star Anise Gummies

These little morsels of joy are so easy to pop into your mouth for a flavour sensation, but are also very soothing for your digestive system, with ingredients that help repair the lining of your gut. Licorice is rich in anti-inflammatory compounds that help suppress pathogenic bacteria. Paired with gelatin, rich in gut-healing amino acids, you have a remedial snack that tastes more like a childhood treat. This recipe is low FODMAP at 4 serves or less.

MAKES 375 ml (12½ fl oz/1½ cups)

340 ml (11½ fl oz/1⅓ cups) cold water
2 tablespoons grass-fed powdered gelatin
1 teaspoon fennel seeds
1 star anise
240 g (8½ oz/2 cups) fresh or frozen raspberries
2 licorice root tea bags
stevia equivalent to 1½ tablespoons of normal sugar

Pour 180 ml (6 fl oz) of the water into a small bowl and sprinkle the gelatin over the surface in an even layer. Set aside for 10 minutes to bloom.

In a medium saucepan, toast the fennel seeds and star anise over a low–medium heat for 30 seconds, or until fragrant. Pour in the remaining 160 ml (5½ fl oz) water, add the raspberries and bring to the boil. Decrease the heat and simmer for 2 minutes. Remove the pan from the heat, add the tea bags and set aside to steep for 3–5 minutes.

Remove the tea bags, squeezing out all of the liquid, and discard.

Add the gelatin mixture and stevia to the hot raspberry liquid and stir until dissolved. Strain through a fine-mesh sieve into a measuring jug, using a spoon to press the raspberry pulp to ensure you get all of the juice out. Don't scrape, as you don't want to push too many of the seeds through. Top up the liquid with water to make 375 ml (12½ fl oz/1½ cups), if necessary.

Place ice cube trays or silicon moulds onto small baking trays. Fill with the raspberry liquid. Refrigerate for at least 1 hour, or until completely set.

To unmould, briefly dip the base of the ice cube trays or moulds into boiling water. Using your fingertips, gently pull the gummies away from the edge of the moulds to release the seal, then invert onto a plate.

Store the gummies in an airtight container in the refrigerator for up to 2 weeks.

CARLA'S TIP These gummies can be made using different mould shapes. The recipe also makes a great layer for a healthy trifle. Just use the Salted Miso Brownies (page 225) as a base layer, add a gummy layer and a layer of coconut yoghurt, then sprinkle with crushed roasted hazelnuts.

Desserts

Raw Blueberry, Lavender & Coconut Cream Flan

What's better than a dessert that doesn't require any cooking? The result looks like haute cuisine, but it's so simple to make and lovely to eat, without any of the bloatedness that often comes with eating sweets. Thanks to the presence of polyphenols, blueberries have a significant anti-inflammatory effect in the body. I've chosen delicious pecans for the base, which a study found rapidly increase antioxidant levels in the bloodstream after eating.

SERVES 8

Base

140 g (5 oz/1 cup) pecans

20 g (¾ oz/¼ cup) unsweetened desiccated (shredded) coconut

80 ml (2½ fl oz/⅓ cup) coconut butter, melted

1 tablespoon extra-virgin coconut oil, melted

1 teaspoon natural vanilla extract

1 teaspoon ground cinnamon

½ teaspoon ground ginger

pinch of sea salt

Filling

80 ml (2½ fl oz/⅓ cup) cold water

1 tablespoon grass-fed powdered gelatin

300 g (10½ oz) blueberries, fresh or frozen & thawed

250 ml (8½ fl oz/1 cup) coconut cream

1 teaspoon natural vanilla extract

1 teaspoon edible (unsprayed) lavender flowers

stevia equal to 1 tablespoon regular sugar

blueberries, pecans, toasted coconut & edible flowers, to garnish

250 g (9 oz/1 cup) coconut yoghurt, to serve (optional)

Lightly grease a 3 cm (1¼ in) deep, 20 cm (8 in) springform tart tin with coconut oil. Refrigerate to set.

To prepare the base, blend all ingredients in a food processor until the mixture begins to bind. Press the mix into the prepared tin to cover the base and sides. Smooth over and compact with the back of a spoon. Refrigerate for 15 minutes, or until firmly set.

Meanwhile, to prepare the filling, pour the cold water into a small bowl and sprinkle the gelatin over the surface in an even layer. Set aside for 10 minutes to bloom.

In a medium saucepan, simmer the blueberries over a low–medium heat for 10 minutes, or until soft and pulpy. Add the gelatin mixture and stir to dissolve. Set aside to cool slightly.

Combine the cooled blueberries, coconut cream, vanilla, lavender and stevia in a high-speed blender and blend until smooth. Pour the filling into the base. Refrigerate for 4 hours, or until firm enough that the surface springs back when pressed.

Decorate the flan with some fresh blueberries, pecans, toasted coconut and edible flowers. Serve with coconut yoghurt, if desired.

Cover and store in the refrigerator for up to 5 days.

CARLA'S TIP Strawberries would work just as well with this recipe, as would blackberries.

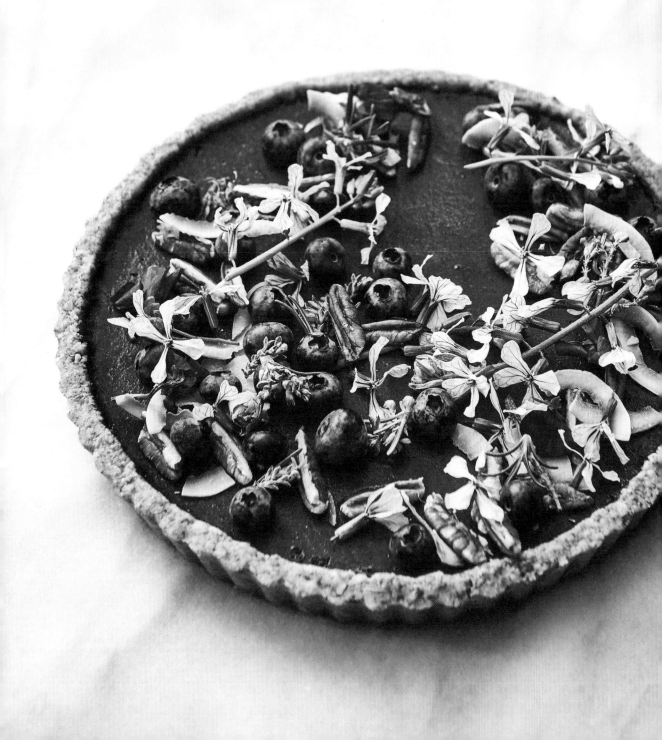

Rhubarb & Pear Cobbler
with Coconut Dumplings

When it comes to comforting desserts, puddings and dumplings are the two that satisfy me most. This warming yet sumptuous dessert is like bread and butter pudding meets apple pie. It should keep your microbial community quite happy too. Fibre-rich rhubarb has traditionally been used to ease abdominal discomfort and constipation. Here it is paired with coconut flour and pear, both great sources of fibre to help keep you regular.

SERVES 6

500 g (1 lb 2 oz, approx. 1 bunch) rhubarb,
    cut into 5 cm (2 in) lengths
500 g (1 lb 2 oz, approx. 3 medium) ripe pears,
    quartered, cored & sliced into thirds lengthways
4 Medjool dates, pitted & coarsely chopped
zest of 1 unwaxed lemon
80 ml (2½ fl oz/⅓ cup) water
4 tablespoons arrowroot
1 tablespoon freshly squeezed lemon juice
2 tablespoons pure organic maple syrup
1 teaspoon natural vanilla extract
½ teaspoon ground cinnamon, plus extra for dusting
100 g (3½ oz/1 cup) ground almonds
40 g (1½ oz/⅓ cup) coconut flour
1 teaspoon gluten-free baking powder
1½ tablespoons unsalted cultured butter,
    chilled & diced
2 free-range organic eggs, lightly beaten
80 ml (2½ fl oz/⅓ cup) tinned coconut milk,
    plus extra for brushing
80 ml (2½ fl oz/⅓ cup) almond milk
coconut yoghurt, to serve (optional)

Preheat the oven to 190°C (375°F/Gas Mark 5).

In a medium bowl, toss the rhubarb, pears, dates and lemon zest. Transfer the mix into a 2 litre (68 fl oz/8 cup) capacity ovenproof dish.

In a small bowl, mix the water and 2 tablespoons of the arrowroot. Add the lemon juice, 1 tablespoon maple syrup, the vanilla and cinnamon. Pour over the fruit and set aside.

In a medium bowl, combine the ground almonds, coconut flour, remaining arrowroot and baking powder and stir. Use your fingers to rub in the butter until it resembles coarse crumbs. In a separate bowl, whisk the eggs, coconut milk, almond milk and the remaining maple syrup. Pour the wet into the dry ingredients and stir until well combined. Set aside for 10 minutes to rehydrate the coconut flour.

Drop six evenly sized lumps of the dumpling mixture over the fruit. Brush with some coconut milk and lightly dust with cinnamon.

Cover the tray with aluminium foil and bake for 30 minutes until the filling is beginning to bubble up around the sides. Remove the foil and bake for a further 15 minutes, or until the dumplings are golden brown. Serve with coconut yoghurt, if desired.

CARLA'S TIP If you don't have pears, you can swap them for apples with their skins on for a prebiotic-rich dessert.

    Gluten Free   Vegetarian   Stage 4 Friendly

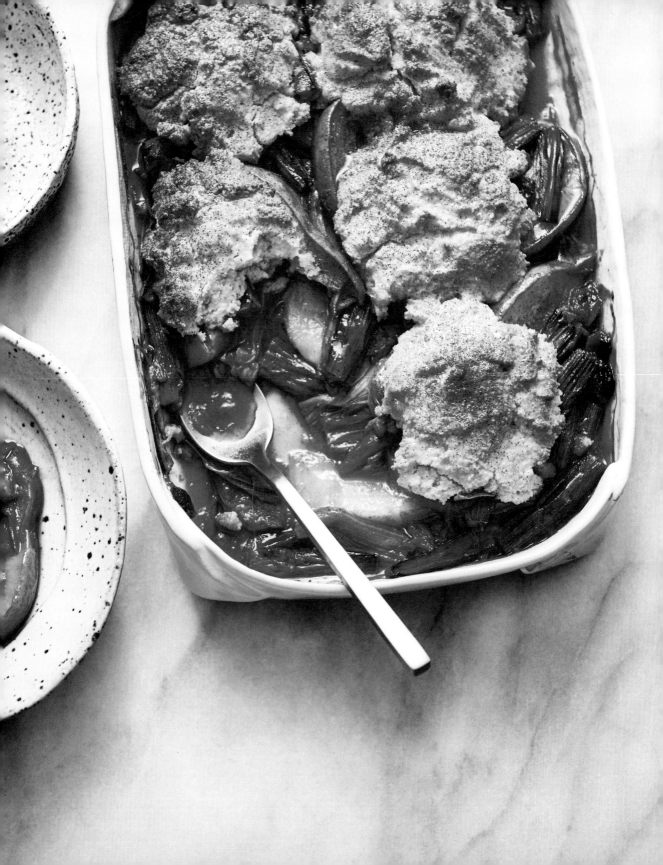

Raspberry Mousse

Image page 214

There is a reason why I always have panna cotta and mousse in my refrigerator. Their special, velvety texture is so soft, soothing and satisfying. I must confess to having them for breakfast as well as dessert, but really, there is no guilt attached as this delicate version with raspberries and rosewater is light, healthy and gut-friendly. Gelatin makes a wonderful thickener and gelling agent and is rich in glycine, an amino acid that plays a vital role in maintaining the mucosal lining of the gut. It also helps balance digestive enzymes, preventing nutrient deficiencies and common gut issues.

SERVES 4 (½ cup capacity moulds)

80 ml (2½ fl oz/⅓ cup) cold water

2 teaspoons grass-fed powdered gelatin

400 ml (13½ fl oz) unsweetened UHT coconut milk

125 g (4½ oz/1 cup) raspberries,
    fresh or frozen & thawed,
    plus extra fresh raspberries to serve

1 tablespoon rosewater (optional)

1 teaspoon natural vanilla extract

stevia equal to 1 tablespoon regular sugar, or to taste

Pour the cold water into a medium heatproof bowl. Sprinkle the gelatin over the surface in an even layer. Set aside for 10 minutes to bloom.

Combine the coconut milk and raspberries in a blender and blend until smooth. Strain through a fine-mesh sieve into a medium bowl. Add the rosewater (if using), vanilla and stevia and stir to combine.

Set the bowl of gelatin over a saucepan of barely simmering water. Gently heat the gelatin, stirring occasionally, until it dissolves. Remove from the heat and gradually pour into the raspberry–coconut mixture, stirring continuously to combine.

Pour the mixture into 125 ml (4 fl oz/½ cup) capacity glasses or containers. Refrigerate for 4 hours, or until set enough that the surface holds its shape when touched.

Serve the mousse topped with fresh raspberries.

CARLA'S TIP Store leftover mousse in the refrigerator for up to 1 week (if it lasts that long). If you are not following a low-FODMAP diet and are in Stage 2 or beyond, you can swap the unsweetened UHT coconut milk for tinned coconut milk and reduce the gelatin to 1½ teaspoons for a richer, creamier mousse.

Desserts

Gluten Free   Dairy Free   Stage 1 Friendly   Low FODMAP

Salted Miso Brownies

Image page 214

This recipe proves that you can have your brownie and eat it too. While the antioxidant powers of cacao powder are well known, studies now show that polyphenol-rich cacao has a prebiotic effect on the gut flora, increasing beneficial bacteria. Miso gives these brownies a delicious salty caramel note, and your gut a biotic boost.

MAKES 16 brownies

250 g (9 oz/2½ cups) ground almonds

80 g (2¾ oz/1 cup) raw cacao powder

30 g (1 oz/¼ cup) arrowroot

1 tablespoon psyllium husk

1 teaspoon gluten-free baking powder

¼ teaspoon bicarbonate of soda (baking soda)

pinch of sea salt flakes, plus extra for sprinkling

180 ml (6 fl oz/¾ cup) drinking coconut milk

125 ml (4 fl oz/½ cup) pure organic maple syrup

100 g (3½ oz) unsalted cultured butter,
    melted & cooled

3 free-range organic eggs

2 tablespoons white miso paste

1 teaspoon natural vanilla extract

1 teaspoon unpasteurised apple-cider vinegar

45 g (1½ oz/⅓ cup) roasted hazelnuts, skins rubbed
    off & coarsely chopped

Preheat the oven to 180°C (350°F/Gas Mark 4). Lightly grease a 20 cm × 20 cm (8 in × 8 in) tray and line with baking paper.

Combine the ground almonds, cacao, arrowroot, psyllium husk, baking powder, bicarb soda and salt in a food processor and blend for 1 minute, or until the mixture resembles flour. Add the coconut milk, maple syrup, butter, eggs, miso, vanilla and vinegar and blend to combine.

Pour the mixture into the prepared tray. Evenly spread and smooth out the surface. Scatter with hazelnuts, sprinkle with sea salt flakes and bake for 25 minutes, or until the surface is set and a skewer comes out clean when inserted into the centre. Set aside to cool completely before cutting the brownie into 16 pieces.

Desserts

CARLA'S TIP If you are avoiding adding natural sugars to your recipes, swap the maple syrup for stevia.

Gluten Free   Vegetarian   Stage 4 Friendly

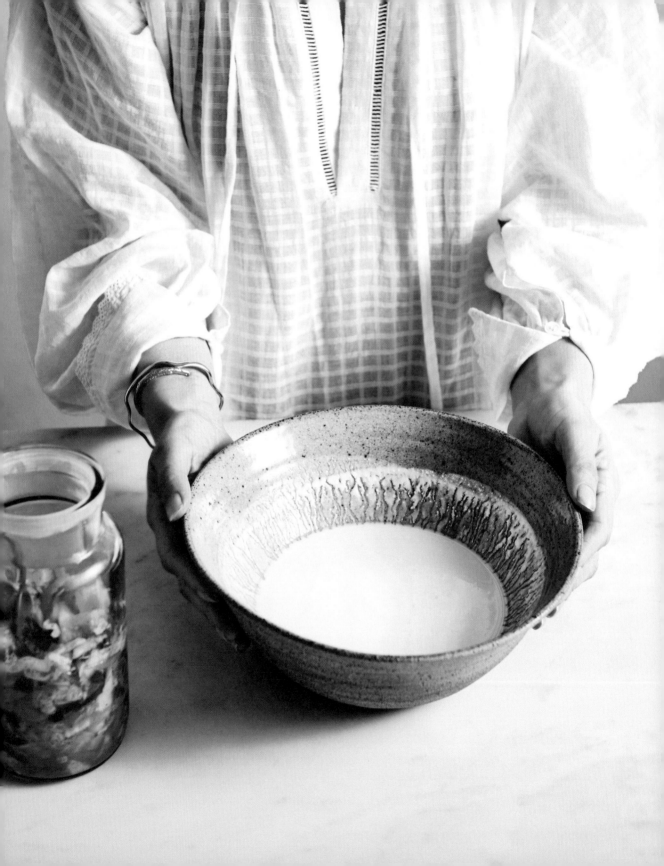

Basics

Coconut Milk Kefir

This is a very popular beverage, with its tangy, yoghurt-like flavours and hint of effervescence, revered in Russia and Eastern Europe for its health benefits. Brimming with beneficial bacteria, this wonder-elixir helps boost digestive, immune and skin health and quashes pathogenic bacteria. Here, we use coconut milk instead of the milk traditionally used in kefir – it works just as well and has more anti-fungal properties.

MAKES 500 ml (17 fl oz/2 cups)

500 ml (17 fl oz/2 cups) organic tinned coconut milk
1 teaspoon coconut sugar
20 g (¾ oz) milk kefir grains (purchased online or sourced from a friend)

Coconut Milk Kefir Grain Storage
1–7 days: In a sterilised glass jar covered with organic cow's milk. Refrigerate.
7–14 days: In a sterilised glass jar with no liquid. Refrigerate.
14+ days (up to 6 months): Dehydrate at room temperature or using a dehydrator set at 30°C (86°F). Freeze in a resealable bag.

Caring for Coconut Milk Kefir Grains
Milk kefir grains – miniature cauliflower-like clumps with a cottage cheese–like texture – are a combination of healthy bacteria and yeast that feed on lactose, the sugars found in milk. As coconut milk does not contain lactose, it is important, after fermenting every second batch of coconut kefir, to feed your grains to aid optimum health. Simply cover the grains with organic cow's milk in a sterilised glass jar. Cover the jar with muslin cloth and secure with a rubber band. Let it stand out at room temperature for 12–24 hours, then strain. For those particularly sensitive to lactose, grains can be rinsed under cold water when transferring from dairy milk to coconut milk.

Pour the coconut milk into a sterilised 750 ml (25½ fl oz/3 cups) capacity glass jar. Add the coconut sugar and grains and stir with a wooden or ceramic spoon. Cover the jar with a muslin cloth and secure with a rubber band. Let it stand at room temperature, out of direct sunlight and in a well-ventilated place, for 12–24 hours, until the coconut milk develops a pleasant, sour taste. Strain through a nonreactive strainer, such as stainless steel or plastic, into a sterilised 500 ml (17 fl oz/2 cup) capacity glass jar or bottle. Reserve the grains, which you can use to begin culturing your next batch of coconut milk kefir, or store them. Seal the jar or bottle and refrigerate for a second ferment of 1–2 days until it's thickened to the consistency of drinking yoghurt. Store the coconut milk kefir in the refrigerator for up to 2 weeks.

CARLA'S TIP The longer you store kefir grains, the longer they take to regain their original fermenting strength. To give them a kick-start, cover with organic cow's milk in a sterilised glass jar, add ½ teaspoon organic raw sugar and stir to combine. Cover the jar with a muslin cloth and secure with a rubber band. Let it stand at room temperature for 12 hours. Strain and repeat 1–3 more times, depending on how long the grains were stored. Coconut Milk Kefir is low FODMAP at 60 ml (2 fl oz/¼ cup) per serve.

Gluten Free   Vegetarian   Vegan   Stage 2 Friendly   Low FODMAP

Bone Broth

Bone broth is a staple in my freezer. Not only is it a flavoursome base for soups and stews, it's also a powerful gut healer. Collagen-rich gelatin, released from the bones during cooking, is an excellent multi-tasker: it nourishes and helps fight inflammation, and is beneficial for restoring the strength of your gut lining. Note, however, that bone broth can be high in histamines, which cause a reaction in some people. If you feel worse after consuming bone broth, histamines may be an issue for you.

MAKES approx. 4 litres (135 fl oz/16 cups)

IDEAL COOKING TIMES

Vegetarian: 1 hour
Fish: 8–12 hours
Chicken: 12–24 hours
Beef & lamb bones: 24–48 hours

1 bunch spring onions (scallions), green part only, roughly chopped
2 carrots, halved crossways
2 celery sticks, halved crossways
2 tablespoons unpasteurised apple-cider vinegar
1 bunch parsley, leaves removed
10 thyme sprigs
1 rosemary stalk (optional)
8 black peppercorns
4 litres (135 fl oz/16 cups) water
1 kg (2 lb 3 oz) bones or 3 tablespoons white miso (for Vegetarian Broth)

Put the vegetables, apple-cider vinegar, herbs and peppercorns in a large stockpot that can hold at least 5 litres (5 quarts) water. Pour in the water and bring to the boil. Reduce to a low heat, add the bones (or miso if you're making vegetarian broth), and simmer according to the cooking instructions on the left. Skim the surface occasionally to remove impurities and excess fat. The broth can also be prepared in a slow cooker.

Strain the broth through a sieve lined with a large coffee filter. If your broth contains a lot of fat, refrigerate overnight to allow the fat to set in a layer on the surface. The following day, scoop out the fat. At this stage, the broth will look like jelly, but once heated, it will become liquid again. Store in the refrigerator for up to 5 days or freeze in 250 ml (8½ fl oz/1 cup) portions for up to 3 months.

CARLA'S TIP You can use chicken, beef, fish or lamb bones. Organic and grass-fed bones are best. The bones can be cooked or uncooked, but if using raw bones, it improves the flavour if you roast them in the oven for around 30 minutes first, especially for beef bones. Aim for 1 kg (2 lb 3 oz) of bones for every 4 litres (135 fl oz/16 cups) of water.

Basics

Kimchi with Daikon, Cabbage & Apple

Eating kimchi is one of the best ways to spice up a meal and promote microbial diversity and robust health at the same time. This Korean recipe, rich in beneficial bacteria and prebiotic fibre, is traditionally served with every meal as a condiment to promote flavour and digestion. It is super easy to create and enhances everything from eggs and soba noodles to soups and fried rice. The aroma is as pungent as the flavour, so keep it well sealed in the refrigerator!

MAKES 1 kg (2 lb 3 oz)

1 kg (2 lb 3 oz, 1 medium) wombok (Chinese) cabbage
600g (1 lb 5 oz, 1 medium) daikon (white radish)
200 g (7 oz, 1 large) green cooking apple
   (such as Granny Smith), cored & quartered
1 litre (34 fl oz/4 cups) water
60 g (2 fl oz/¼ cup) sea salt

Kimchi Paste
5 spring onions (scallions), white part only,
   finely chopped
25 g (1 oz/¼ cup) Korean chilli powder
   (kochukaru/gochugaru)
60 ml (2 fl oz/¼ cup) tamari
2 tablespoons fish sauce (optional)
5 cloves garlic, finely chopped
3 tablespoons finely grated ginger

Remove and reserve the outer leaves of the cabbage, then trim the base. Cut lengthways into quarters, then crossways at approximately 5 cm (2 in) intervals. Wash thoroughly and drain, then put the cabbage into a large ceramic or glass bowl.

Using a mandolin, thinly slice the daikon into rounds, followed by the apple. Add to the bowl with the cabbage.

Combine the water and salt in a jug or bowl, stirring to dissolve the salt to make a brine. Pour the brine over the vegetables.

Wearing food handling gloves, or with clean hands, massage the brine into the vegetables for 1–2 minutes until they soften. Cover with the reserved cabbage leaves and weigh down with a plate so the vegetables are submerged in brine. Cover with muslin cloth and secure with a rubber band or some string. Set aside at room temperature, in a well ventilated place and out of direct sunlight, for at least 8 hours or overnight.

Remove and reserve the top cabbage leaves. Drain the vegetables, reserving 250 ml (8½ fl oz/ 1 cup) of brine. Put the vegetables in a large bowl.

CARLA'S TIP Nutritious kimchi juice can be used to make a delicious virgin Bloody Mary or as a dressing on noodles or to spice up soups.

Gluten Free   Dairy Free   Vegetarian Option   Vegan Option   Stage 3 Friendly

To prepare the kimchi paste, combine the spring onion, Korean chilli powder, tamari, fish sauce (if using), garlic and ginger in a small bowl and stir well.

Wearing food handling gloves, or with clean hands, massage the paste into the vegetables for 1–2 minutes until they begin to release liquid to form a brine.

Tightly pack the mixture into a sterilised 1.5–2 litre (6–8 cup) capacity glass jar, or use a ceramic fermentation crock with a water seal if you have one. Firmly press the vegetables down to submerge them under the brine, adding the reserved brine to top up if required. Cover with the reserved cabbage leaves and weigh down with a ceramic weight or small jar filled with water to ensure the vegetables stay submerged. Ensure there is a 5 cm (2 in) gap between the cabbage leaves and the top of the jar to allow for extra liquid released during the fermentation process. Place on a large plate to catch any overflow liquid. If using a glass jar, cover with a double layer of muslin cloth and secure with a rubber band. If using a specialised ceramic fermentation crock, half-fill the water seal trough with water and cover with the lid. Remember to refill the water trough over the fermentation period as required.

Set aside at room temperature, in a well ventilated place and out of direct sunlight, for at least 5–7 days (depending on the temperature of your kitchen – warmth speeds up the process), or until the liquid increases and you start to see little bubbles, the vegetables shrivel up and the mixture becomes pleasantly tangy. Check daily to ensure the vegetables are completely submerged in brine to prevent mould from forming. Press down the weight and refill the water seal trough if using a specialised ceramic fermentation crock as required.

Kimchi can be used immediately. Store in the refrigerator for up to 1 year.

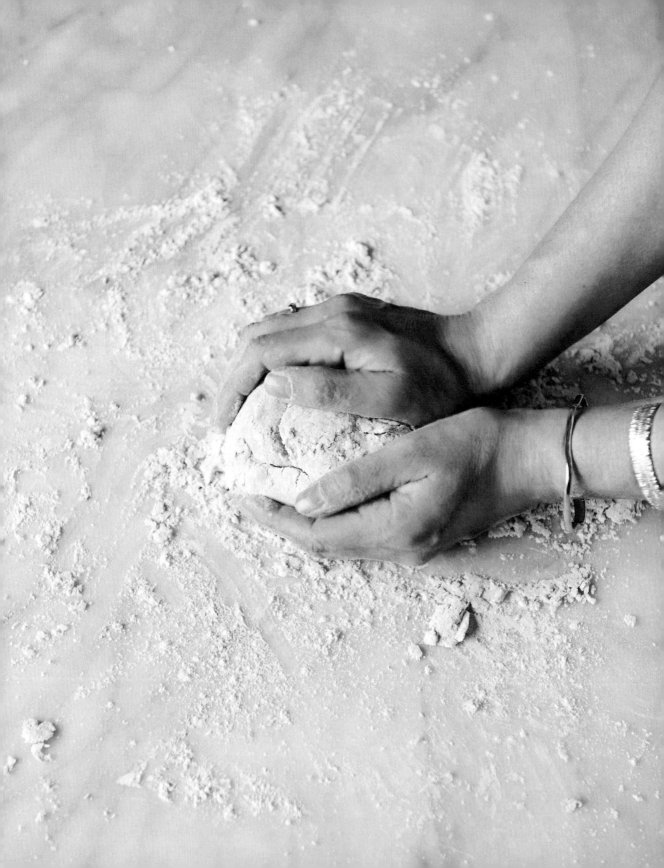

Buckwheat Pasta

I love traditional pasta, but unfortunately my microbiome doesn't. I've come up with a lovely recipe that keeps us both very happy. It can be used to make all types of pastas, from pappardelle and fettuccine to agnolotti. The beauty of buckwheat is that, contrary to its name, it's actually wheat- and gluten-free, making it the perfect pasta alternative for sensitive tummies. It is also an excellent, plant-based source of protein and fibre, and according to recent research may increase the activity of our antioxidant pathways, reducing both oxidative stress and inflammation in the body. Psyllium husk can be harsh on the digestive tract for some, while for others it helps keep things regular. I use it in small amounts (it's allowed on a low-FODMAP diet); here, it acts as a helpful binding agent.

SERVES 4

125 ml (4 fl oz/½ cup) water
1½ tablespoons psyllium husk
2 free-range organic eggs
1 tablespoon extra-virgin olive oil,
    plus extra for drizzling
225 g (8 oz/1½ cups) buckwheat flour
90 g (3 oz/¾ cup) arrowroot
½ teaspoon sea salt

Dusting Flour
35 g (1¼ oz/¼ cup) buckwheat flour
2 tablespoons arrowroot

To make the dusting flour, combine the ingredients in a small bowl and set aside.

To make the pasta, combine the water and psyllium husk in a small bowl. Set aside for 3 minutes to thicken into a gel-like liquid. Add the eggs and oil and whisk to combine.

In a medium bowl, whisk the flour, arrowroot and salt. Add the psyllium mixture and stir to form a rough dough. Turn it out onto a clean bench and knead for 5 minutes, or until smooth. Shape the dough into a rectangle, wrap in plastic wrap and refrigerate for 15 minutes.

Cover a clean bench with the dusting flour. Separate the dough into quarters. Roll out, one at a time, very thinly, into 30 cm × 20 cm (12 in × 8 in) rectangles, dusting with buckwheat flour as necessary to prevent sticking. Keep the remaining dough covered to prevent drying out.

For fettuccine, cut lengthways into 1 cm (½ in) thick strips. For pappardelle, cut lengthways into 2 cm (¾ in) thick strips. For agnolotti, use a 10 cm (4 in) round cookie cutter to stamp out discs.

To cook the pasta, bring a large saucepan of water to the boil. Add the pasta, stirring once or twice, for 3–4 minutes, or until al dente and just tender.

Drain and drizzle the pasta with extra-virgin olive oil, tossing to coat and to prevent sticking or clumping. Eat immediately.

CARLA'S TIP For a quick, simple vegetarian pasta, warm some Pumpkin Seed & Herb Pesto (page 244) with a generous splash of tinned coconut milk to make a creamy herbaceous sauce, or stir through some Nut-Free Roasted Romesco (page 241).

Turmeric Roti

Roti is a delicious traditional Indian flatbread. It makes a wonderful accompaniment to curries and eggs, and can also be used as a wrap for lunches. This gluten-free version boasts the benefits of anti-inflammatory turmeric. This spice is known for its healing qualities: studies have shown that curcumin (the natural polyphenolic compound responsible for its vibrant orange colour) may have regulative effects on the gut microbiota and may help to repair the stomach lining. I've included black pepper in this recipe too, as it helps increase the bioavailability of turmeric.

MAKES 8

140 g (5 oz/1 cup) white rice flour
½ teaspoon sea salt
½ teaspoon ground turmeric
¼ teaspoon finely ground black pepper
2 organic eggs
250 ml (8½ fl oz/1 cup) water
2 teaspoons ghee, melted & cooled,
    or extra-virgin olive oil, plus extra for greasing

In a medium bowl, whisk the rice flour, salt, turmeric and black pepper. In a separate bowl, whisk the eggs, water and ghee. Add the wet to the dry ingredients, whisking until well combined.

Cover the bowl and refrigerate for 1 hour.

Preheat a 20 cm (8 in) cast-iron or non-stick frying pan over a medium–high heat. Wipe with paper towel dipped in ghee to very lightly grease.

Whisk the rested roti batter, then pour 60 ml (2 fl oz/¼ cup) into the centre of the pan, quickly swirling to create an even layer. Cook the roti for 30–60 seconds, or until the surface dries out and small holes appear. Flip and cook for a further 20 seconds, or until golden.

Transfer the roti to a plate, cover with a clean tea towel (dish towel) to keep warm, and set aside. Repeat with the remaining batter.

Wrap the cooled roti in plastic wrap and store in the refrigerator for up to 1 week. Alternatively, lay some baking paper between each roti, wrap in plastic wrap and freeze for up to 3 months.

    Gluten Free   Dairy Free   Vegetarian   Stage 2 Friendly   Low FODMAP

Low-FODMAP Charcoal Flatbread

There is something very satisfying about this savoury, healthful bread; as you eat it, you know it is doing you good. Activated charcoal binds to and helps eliminate toxins in the stomach. A study published in the American Journal of Gastroenterology *found that activated charcoal, when taken before or after a meal, can reduce gas, bloating and stomach cramps. Eliminating toxins and harmful bacteria is of particular importance while healing the gut, which is why I came up with this FODMAP-friendly, allergen-free flatbread perfect for any stage of the Gut Guide, and particularly for Stage 1.*

SERVES 6

65 g (2¼ oz/⅓ cup) buckwheat groats
1 tablespoon unpasteurised apple-cider vinegar,
    plus a splash for soaking
225 g (8 oz/1½ cups) buckwheat flour
60 g (2 oz/½ cup) arrowroot
2 teaspoons gluten-free baking powder
2 teaspoons activated charcoal powder
1 teaspoon sea salt, plus extra for sprinkling
½ teaspoon bicarbonate of soda (baking soda)
300 ml (10 fl oz/1¼ cups) almond milk
2 teaspoons extra-virgin olive oil, plus extra
    for brushing

CARLA'S TIP Charcoal can dry out the bread quite quickly, so it is best eaten fresh on the day of baking. Alternatively, store immediately in an airtight container in the refrigerator for up to 4 days, toasting or warming it up in the microwave to soften it.

Fill a small bowl halfway with warm water. Add the buckwheat groats and a splash of apple-cider vinegar and set aside in a warm place to soak for at least 2 (and up to 6) hours. Drain and rinse.

Sift the buckwheat flour, arrowroot, baking powder, charcoal powder, salt and bicarb soda into a large mixing bowl. Add the buckwheat groats and mix to combine.

In a separate bowl, whisk the almond milk, apple-cider vinegar and oil. Pour the mix into the dry ingredients and stir with a wooden spoon until well combined. Cover with a tea towel (dish towel) and allow the dough to rest for approximately 1 hour. By then it should have absorbed any excess liquid, but the consistency should still be sticky to the touch.

Preheat the oven to 200°C (400°F/Gas Mark 6). Line a baking tray with baking paper.

Place the dough on the baking tray and use the back of a spoon to smooth it out into a 20 cm × 30 cm (8 in × 12 in) rectangular shape, approximately 1 cm (½ in) thick. Brush the surface generously with olive oil. Sprinkle with some sea salt, then bake in the oven for 15–20 minutes, or until the dough has risen slightly and is springy to the touch.

Allow to cool for 5 minutes before slicing.

Basics

Sauerkraut with Carrot, Caraway Seeds & Juniper Berries

Fermentation is a completely natural biological process that is also pure genius, as it creates bio-active, medicinal foods with immune-modulating and anti-inflammatory properties. Fermented fare is the ultimate synbiotic – prebiotic, probiotic, postbiotic. It is rich in enzymes that help break down hard-to-digest proteins, making it perfect as a condiment with meals. The age-old art of fermentation yields so many health benefits for your gut, immune, metabolic and skin health, and fermented foods are so easy to make. To enhance this recipe's gut-loving properties, I've added gut-calming caraway seeds and antioxidant-rich juniper berries.

MAKES Approx. 4 cups

1 kg (2 lb 3 oz/1 medium) red or green cabbage, outer
    leaves removed & reserved
2 tablespoons sea salt
2 large carrots, coarsely grated
1 large handful dill, coarsely chopped
1 tablespoon caraway seeds, lightly toasted
10 juniper berries

Cut the cabbage in half, then remove and discard the core. Thinly shred, wash and drain, then put in a large glass or ceramic bowl. Add the salt and massage into the cabbage for 2–3 minutes to release its liquid and to soften. The salt will combine with that liquid to form a brine. Add the carrots, dill, caraway seeds and berries and toss to combine.

Tightly pack the mixture into a sterilised 1.5 litre (6 cup) glass jar, earthenware fermentation crockpot or specialised fermentation jar with an airtight lid. Pour the brine over the top and firmly press the vegetables down to submerge. Cover with the reserved cabbage leaves.

Weigh down the mixture using a specialised ceramic weight or small jar filled with water to keep the contents submerged (if you are using a jar with an airtight lid, there's no need). Ensure there is a 5 cm (2 in) gap between the cabbage and the top of the jar to allow for extra liquid released during fermentation. If you're using a glass jar,

cover with a double layer of muslin (cheese cloth) and secure with a rubber band. If using a crockpot or jar, secure the lid.

Let stand at room temperature, out of direct sunlight and in a well ventilated place, for 1–2 weeks, or until the kraut smells and tastes sour. The length of time will vary depending on the temperature of your kitchen. During this time, if using a jar covered with muslin, check daily to ensure the vegetables are completely submerged in brine.

Sauerkraut can be used immediately or stored in the refrigerator for a week to age before use.

CARLA'S TIP Once fermented, you can transfer your sauerkraut into smaller sterilised jars. Make sure to pack the jars tightly to submerge everything in brine and seal with a lid. The sauerkraut can be stored in the refrigerator for up to 3 months – the flavours will continue to develop.

LOW-FODMAP OPTION People who are low FODMAP can enjoy sauerkraut made with red cabbage at 75 g (2¾ oz) per serve.

     Gluten Free   Dairy Free   Vegetarian   Vegan   Stage 3 Friendly   Low-FODMAP Option

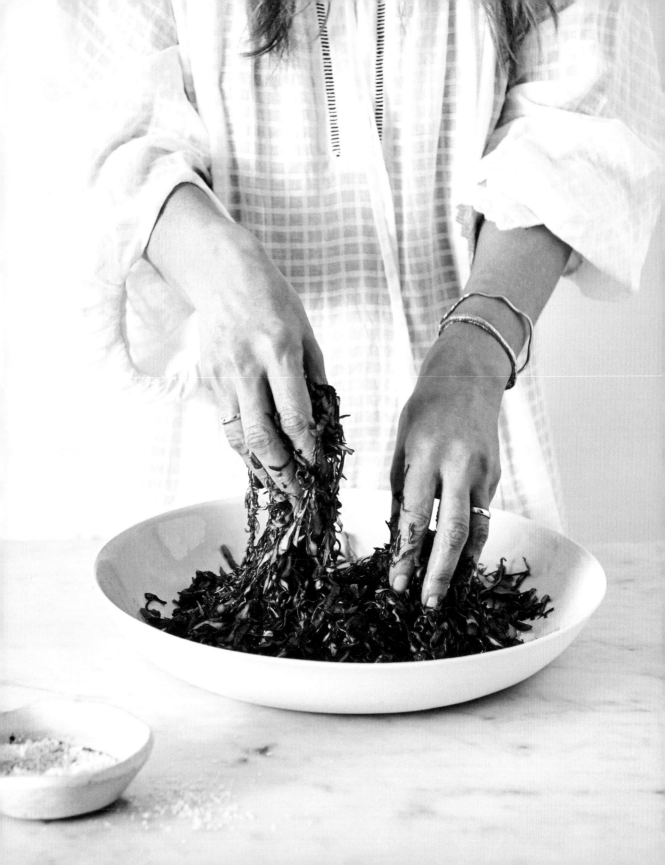

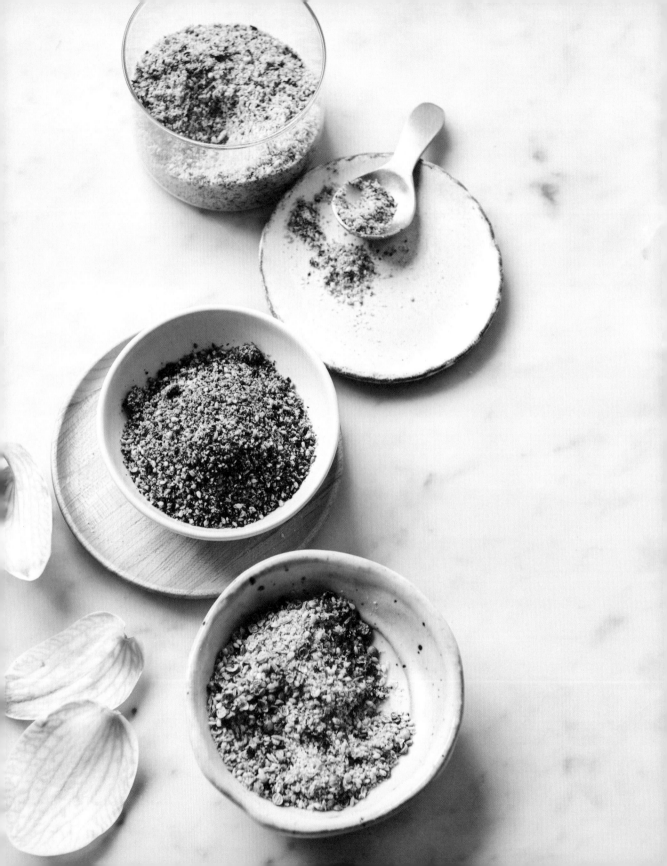

Sesame Salt, Three Ways

Homemade sauces, salts and sauerkraut are staples in my kitchen, and are very handy whenever I am tired and want something simple but flavoursome. They can embellish a piece of fish, chicken or a baked sweet potato. These seasonings also give meals a powerful digestive kick. Coriander seeds work like an antispasmodic, relaxing digestive muscles and easing the discomfort of irritable bowel syndrome and other gut disorders, while fennel seeds help kick-start digestion. Adding a healthy source of fats such as sesame seeds to a nutrient-dense meal can aid in the absorption of fat-soluble vitamins such as vitamin E, which is important for its protective antioxidant activity. Sprinkle the below combinations over your salads and meals as a spiced-up alternative to salt.

MAKES Approx. 100 g (3½ oz/¾ cup)

Coriander, Chilli & Fennel
2 teaspoons coriander seeds
½ teaspoon dried chilli flakes
1 teaspoon fennel seeds
75 g (2¾ oz/½ cup) white sesame seeds
2 teaspoons sea salt

Matcha
35 g (1¼ oz/¼ cup) each black & white sesame seeds
2 teaspoons sea salt
2 teaspoons matcha (green tea) powder

Goma-shio
2 teaspoons sea salt
10 g (¼ oz/⅓ cup) dried instant wakame flakes
75 g (2¾ oz/½ cup) white sesame seeds

For the Coriander, Chilli & Fennel, toast all ingredients in a medium frying pan over a low heat for 10 minutes, or until golden and fragrant. Stir occasionally to ensure the seeds do not burn. Set aside to cool. Coarsely grind using a mortar and pestle, spice grinder or food processor.

For the Matcha, toast the black and white sesame seeds and salt in a medium frying pan over a low heat, tossing occasionally, for 5 minutes, or until golden. Set aside to cool. Once cooled, add the matcha powder and coarsely grind using a mortar and pestle, spice grinder or food processor.

For the Goma-shio, toast the salt and wakame in a medium frying pan over a low heat for 3–4 minutes, or until crisp. Add the sesame seeds and toast, tossing occasionally, for 5 minutes, or until golden. Coarsely grind using a mortar and pestle, spice grinder or food processor.

CARLA'S TIP I've added wakame to my version of Goma-shio sesame salt, a seaweed that contains enzymes needed to help break down heavy starches such as those found in grains, potatoes and beans. It allows them to be more easily digested, making this seasoning a great addition to any grain-based or legume dish. Sesame salts are low-FODMAP at 1 tablespoon (or less) per serve.

Basics

Gluten Free   Dairy Free   Vegetarian   Vegan   Stage 4 Friendly   Low FODMAP

Carrot Noodles

Carrots are low FODMAP and, according to Monash University, can be eaten freely. They contain pro-vitamin A, pectin and polyphenols, which makes them an excellent food to promote gut health. Carrot noodles are a great alternative to pasta, and carrots are very versatile – you can spiralise them (as in this recipe), bake or sauté them.

SERVES 4

750 g (1 lb 11 oz, about 4 large) carrots
sea salt & freshly ground black pepper, to taste
extra-virgin olive oil, for drizzling

Using a spiraliser or peeler, peel the carrots into ribbons or noodles. Blanch in boiling water for 40–60 seconds, or until cooked, but still with a slight bite.

Drain and season with salt and pepper and drizzle with oil. Use as a simple base for Stage 1 of the program, or use instead of cauliflower rice in other recipes for a low-FODMAP alternative.

CARLA'S TIP In Stage 4 enjoy these noodles as a raw salad, dressed simply with extra-virgin olive oil and lemon juice.

Cauliflower Rice

The beauty of cauliflower is that it complements the flavours of whatever you pair it with. Here, I've kept it simple with classic flavours – ghee, onion and garlic – making it a versatile side dish to suit just about any recipe in this book.

SERVES 4 (Makes 800 g/1 lb 2 oz/6 cups)

800 g (1 lb 12 oz/approx. 1 head) cauliflower, cut into
    small florets, stalk coarsely chopped
2 tablespoons ghee or extra-virgin olive oil
1 small onion, finely diced (optional)
1 small garlic clove, finely chopped (optional)
sea salt & freshly ground black pepper, to taste

Blend the cauliflower in a food processor until it forms rice-sized grains.

Heat the ghee in a large frying pan over a medium heat. Cook the onion and garlic until softened, about 1 minute. Add the cauliflower and cook, stirring occasionally, for 5–6 minutes, until just tender and heated through. Season with salt and pepper to serve.

LOW-FODMAP OPTION Some recipes in this book use cauliflower rice as a side. If you are following a low-FODMAP diet, swap for quinoa, white basmati rice or buckwheat.

Basics

Nut-Free Roasted Romesco

This sauce is rich in the alluring and deeply smoky flavours of roasted, spiced red capsicum (bell pepper). Not only is this vegetable one of the highest in vitamin C, it is also a good source of flavonoids, capsaicinoids and phenolic acids, full of anti-inflammatory and antioxidant activity. They help protect the body from free radicals, which cause premature ageing. I always have a batch ready in my refrigerator to spice up a piece of fish, pasta, eggs, baked leeks or brussels sprouts.

MAKES Approx. 750 ml (25½ fl oz/3 cups)

600 g (1 lb 5 oz/about 2 large) red capsicum
    (bell pepper), roughly chopped
300 g (10½ oz) peeled Japanese pumpkin (squash),
    cut into 4 cm (1½ in) chunks
180 g (6½ oz/about 1 medium) carrot,
    cut into 2 cm (¾ in) dice
2 tablespoons extra-virgin olive oil
½ teaspoon sea salt
freshly ground black pepper, to taste
1 teaspoon smoked paprika
¼ teaspoon ground chilli
125 ml (4 fl oz/¼ cup) water

Preheat the oven to 200°C (400°F/Gas Mark 6). Line a baking tray with baking paper.

Toss the capsicum, pumpkin, carrot and olive oil in a bowl to combine. Add the salt, pepper and spices and toss until evenly coated. Spread the vegetables out on the baking tray and roast for 25 minutes, or until softened and caramelised.

Remove from the oven and allow to cool slightly. Blitz the vegetables and water in a blender until smooth.

Transfer the sauce to a sterilised glass bottle or jar and store in the refrigerator for up to 1 week, or in the freezer for up to 2 months.

Basics

CARLA'S TIP Make a big batch and freeze portions in small airtight containers so you always have it on hand. In the later stages of the Gut Guide, when we introduce more nuts, you can make this sauce the more traditional way by adding almonds and/or hazelnuts.

Prebiotic Superseed Bread

This delicious loaf is gluten free and low FODMAP (at two slices per serve), with an extra protein and antioxidant-rich boost from sunflower kernels and pumpkin seeds (pepitas). Your microbes will love it too, with fibre-rich buckwheat paired with the prebiotic power of marshmallow root (which you should be able to find at health food stores). Anti-inflammatory turmeric gives your loaf a rich golden hue!

MAKES 1 Loaf

3 teaspoons sea salt

120 g (4 oz/¾ cup) pumpkin seeds (pepitas), plus extra for topping

65 g (2¼ oz/⅓ cup) buckwheat groats, plus extra for topping

2 teaspoons unpasteurised apple-cider vinegar, plus a splash for soaking

115 g (4 oz/1 cup) arrowroot

150 g (5½ oz/1 cup) buckwheat flour

45 g (1½ oz/¼ cup) chia seeds

2 teaspoons gluten-free baking powder

1 tablespoon ground turmeric

1 tablespoon ground marshmallow root (optional)

1 teaspoon freshly ground black pepper

375 ml (12½ fl oz/1½ cups) water

1 tablespoon extra-virgin olive oil

1 tablespoon sunflower kernels, for topping

Fill a medium bowl three-quarters of the way with warm water. Add 1½ teaspoons of the salt and stir until mostly dissolved. Add the pumpkin seeds, cover the bowl with a clean tea towel (dish towel) and set aside in a warm place to soak for at least 7 (and up to 12) hours. Drain and rinse.

Fill a small bowl halfway with warm water. Add the buckwheat groats and a splash of apple-cider vinegar and set aside in a warm place to soak for 2 (and up to 6) hours. Drain and rinse.

In a large mixing bowl, combine the arrowroot, buckwheat flour, chia seeds, baking powder, turmeric, marshmallow root (if using), soaked seeds, buckwheat groats, pepper and the remaining salt and mix well.

In a separate bowl, whisk the water, oil and apple-cider vinegar. Pour into the dry ingredients and stir with a wooden spoon until well combined. Cover the bowl with a tea towel and allow the dough to rest for approximately 1 hour. Check to ensure the dough has absorbed any excess water, yet still feels wet and sticky to the touch.

Preheat the oven to 180°C (350°F/Gas Mark 4). Lightly grease and line an 18 cm × 8 cm (7 in × 3¼ in) loaf tin with baking paper. Pour the dough into the prepared tin and smooth out the top with the back of a spoon to remove any air bubbles. Sprinkle with sunflower kernels and buckwheat groats, pushing them into the top of the dough. Bake for 1 hour and 10 minutes, or until a skewer comes out clean when inserted into the centre of the bread.

Remove the loaf from the oven, cover with a clean tea towel and let stand for 10 minutes to cool slightly. Turn out onto a rack to cool completely, then slice into 10–12 slices.

Store in an airtight container in the refrigerator for up to 1 week or slice into portions and freeze in reusable bags for up to 3 months.

CARLA'S TIP This bread is great toasted with Miso Probiotic Butter (page 245).

Gluten Free   Dairy Free   Vegetarian   Vegan   Stage 3 Friendly   Low FODMAP

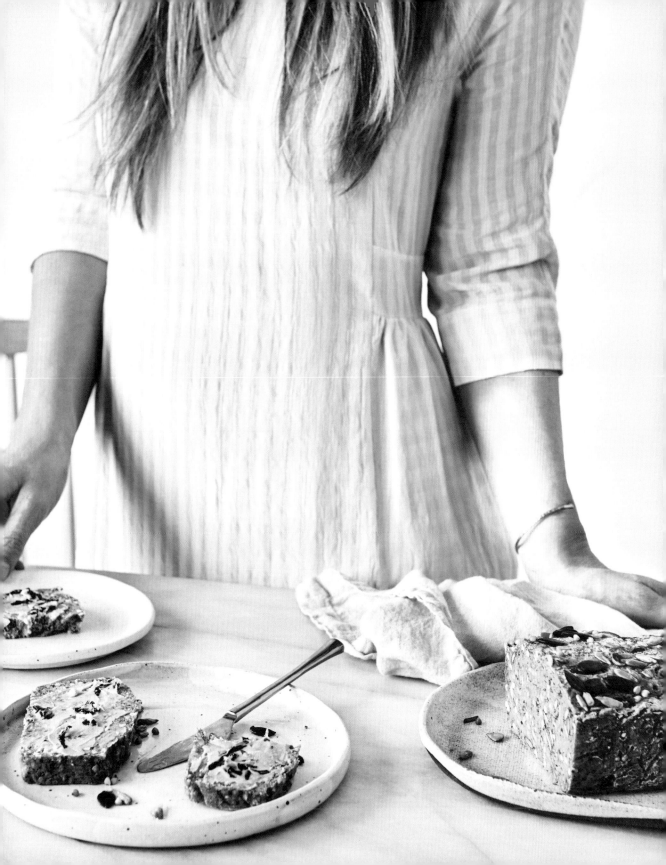

Pumpkin Seed & Herb Pesto

Pesto is a non-negotiable in my house, and it makes last-minute cooking seamless. I pop it on the kids' eggs for breakfast, mix it with pasta for a quick dinner, or smear it on avocado toast, chicken or fish. I've swapped pine nuts for pumpkin seeds, and not just for their earthy flavour. They are anti-parasitic and high in insoluble fibre, and their abundance of zinc makes them great for boosting your immune system and digestive health.

MAKES Approx. 310 g (11 oz/1¼ cups)

1½ teaspoons sea salt
120 g (4½ oz/¾ cup) pumpkin seeds (pepitas)
3 tablespoons nutritional yeast flakes
60 ml (2 fl oz/¼ cup) freshly squeezed lemon juice
zest of 1 unwaxed lemon
4 garlic cloves, peeled
3 large handfuls basil
1 small handful mint
1 large handful flat-leaf (Italian) parsley leaves
1 large handful oregano
125 ml (4 fl oz/½ cup) extra-virgin olive oil,
    plus extra for drizzling
sea salt & freshly ground black pepper, to taste

Fill a medium bowl three-quarters with warm water. Add the salt and stir until mostly dissolved. Add the pumpkin seeds and cover the bowl with a clean tea towel (dish towel). Set aside in a warm place to soak for least 7 (and up to 12) hours. Drain and rinse.

Blend the seeds, yeast flakes, lemon juice and zest and garlic in a small food processor until finely chopped. Add the herbs and, with the motor running, gradually pour in the oil until combined. Season with salt and pepper to taste.

Use immediately or store in an airtight container in the refrigerator for up to 1 week, covering the pesto with a thin layer of olive oil to prevent discolouration.

CARLA'S TIP This pesto contains an amazing 22 g (¾ oz) of fibre. Eat it with carrot sticks for a fibre-rich afternoon snack, or turn it into a salad dressing by adding equal measures of lemon juice and extra-virgin olive oil, to taste.

LOW-FODMAP OPTION To make this recipe low FODMAP, omit the garlic. This pesto is low FODMAP at 62 g (2 oz/¼ cup) per serve.

Gluten Free   Dairy Free   Vegetarian   Vegan   Stage 3 Friendly   Low-FODMAP Option

Miso, Tahini & Umeboshi Dressing

Gluten Free
Vegetarian

DairyFree
Stage 2 Friendly

This delightful dressing brightens everything from baked vegetables and soba noodles to falafel and salads. It is bursting with healthfulness, featuring miso (rich in beneficial phytonutrients), which studies show may help control blood pressure, inflammation and oxidative stress; tahini, which has a high vitamin E content that may help improve intestinal barrier function; and gut-loving umeboshi plums, which infuse a wonderful tartness into the sweet and nutty notes of the dressing.

MAKES Approx. 250 ml (8½ fl oz/1 cup)

60 ml (2 fl oz/¼ cup) tahini, hulled or unhulled
2 tablespoons freshly squeezed lemon juice
1 tablespoon shiro (white) miso paste
1 umeboshi salted plum, seeded & finely chopped
2 teaspoons fresh ginger, finely grated
2 teaspoons manuka honey
60 ml (2 fl oz/¼ cup) water

In a medium bowl, whisk the tahini, lemon juice, miso, umeboshi plum, ginger and honey. Gradually pour in the water, whisking to incorporate and form a smooth dressing.

CARLA'S TIP If you can't get your hands on umeboshi plum, simply omit it and season the dressing with a little sea salt.

Probiotic Butter, Two Ways

Gluten Free
Stage 3 Friendly

Vegetarian
Low FODMAP

Cultured butter is rich and decadent in flavour, yet it is full of the anti-inflammatory fatty acid butyrate. It also contains lactic acid–producing bacteria that help break down lactose (milk sugar) and casein (milk proteins), aiding digestion. Here are two probiotic-boosted versions – one using wakame and miso and the other using antioxidant-rich matcha.

MAKES Approx. 150 g (5½ oz)

Miso & Wakame Butter
150 g (5½ oz) salted cultured butter, diced,
    at room temperature
60 g (2 oz/¼ cup) shiro (white) miso paste
2 tablespoons dried instant wakame flakes

Matcha, Ginger & Kaffir Lime Butter
150 g (5½ oz) salted cultured butter, diced,
    at room temperature
1 teaspoon matcha powder
1 tablespoon fresh ginger, finely grated
2 kaffir lime leaves, de-veined & finely shredded

Beat the butter and miso or matcha in a medium bowl until smooth. Refrigerate for 15 minutes, or until firmed up slightly. Add the wakame or ginger and kaffir lime to the butter mixture and stir to combine. Shape into an 8 cm (3¼ in) log and wrap in baking paper. Roll on the benchtop to form a uniform log, twisting and tightening both ends. Secure the ends. Refrigerate for at least 1 hour until firm enough to slice, or until required.

Store the butter in the refrigerator for up to 1 month or freeze for up to 3 months.

CARLA'S TIP I love to use these butters when baking fish or chicken, as a topping for steamed veggies or even as a creamy addition to soup.

Basics

Reference List

1 Riiser, A 'The Human Microbiome, Asthma, and Allergy.' *Allergy, Asthma, and Clinical Immunology*, (2015) 11:35.

2 Lammers, KM et al. 'Gliadin Induces an Increase in Intestinal Permeability and Zonulin Release by Binding to the Chemokine Receptor CXCR3.' *Gastroenterology*, (2008) 135(1):194–204.

3 Yoon MY and Yoon SS 'Disruption of the Gut Ecosystem by Antibiotics.' *Yonsei Medical Journal*, (2018) 59(1):4–12.

Francino MP 'Antibiotics and the Human Gut Microbiome: Dysbioses and Accumulation of Resistances.' *Frontiers in Microbiology*, (2015) 6:1543.

Langdon A et al. 'The Effects of Antibiotics on the Microbiome throughout Development and Alternative Approaches for Therapeutic Modulation.' *Genome Medicine*, (2016) 8:39.

4 Gareau, MG et al. 'Pathophysiological Mechanisms of Stress-Induced Intestinal Damage.' *Current Molecular Medicine*, (2008) 8(4): 274–281.

5 Huang, YJ 'Asthma Microbiome Studies and the Potential for New Therapeutic Strategies.' *Current Allergy and Asthma Reports*, (2013) 13(5):453–461.

6 Ege, MJ et al. 'Exposure to Environmental Microorganisms and Childhood Asthma.' *New England Journal of Medicine*, (2011) 364:701–709.

7 Campbell, B et al. 'The Effects of Growing Up on a Farm on Adult Lung Function and Allergic Phenotypes: An International Population-Based Study.' *Thorax*, (2017) 72(3):236–244.

8 Mosca, A et al. 'Gut Microbiota Diversity and Human Diseases: Should We Reintroduce Key Predators in Our Ecosystem?' *Frontiers in Microbiology*, (2016) 7:455.

9 De Filippo, C et al. 'Impact of Diet in Shaping Gut Microbiota Revealed by a Comparative Study in Children From Europe and Rural Africa.' *Proceedings of the National Academy of Sciences of the United States of America*, (2010) 107(33): 14691–14696.

10 Ianiro G et al. 'Digestive Enzyme Supplementation in Gastrointestinal Diseases.' *Current Drug Metabolism*, (2016) 17(2):187-93.

11 University of Chicago Medical Center. 'Specific Bacteria in the Small Intestine are Crucial for Fat Absorption.' *ScienceDaily*, (2018). Retrieved from http://www.sciencedaily.com/

12 Menni, C et al. 'Omega-3 Fatty Acids Correlate with Gut Microbiome Diversity and Production of N-Carbamylglutamate in Middle Aged and Elderly Women.' *Scientific Reports*, (2017) 7(1).

13 Antvorskov, JC et al. 'Dietary Gluten Alters the Balance of Pro-Inflammatory and Anti-Inflammatory Cytokines in T Cells of BALB/c Mice.' *Immunology*, (2013) 138(1):23-33.

14 Pruimboom, L and De Punder, K 'The Opioid Effects of Gluten Exorphins: Asymptomatic Celiac Disease.' *Journal of Health, Population, and Nutrition*, (2015) 33:24.

15 He, M et al. 'Effects of Cow's Milk Beta-Casein Variants on Symptoms of Milk Intolerance in Chinese Adults: A Multicentre, Randomised Controlled Study.' *Nutrition Journal*, (2017) 16(1):72.

16 Baker, JM et al. 'Estrogen-Gut Microbiome Axis: Physiological and Clinical Implications.' *Maturitas*, (2017) 103:45–53.

17 LaRue, A 'Xenoestrogens – What Are They? How to Avoid Them.' Women in Balance Institute, (n.d.). Retrieved from http://womeninbalance.org/

18 Caricilli AM and Saad MJ 'The Role of Gut Microbiota on Insulin Resistance.' *Nutrients*, (2013) 5(3):829-51.

19 Kobyliak, N et al. 'Probiotics in Prevention and Treatment of Obesity: A Critical View.' *Nutrition & Metabolism*, (2016) 13:14.

20 Wang, S et al. 'Novel Insights of Dietary Polyphenols and Obesity.' *The Journal of Nutritional Biochemistry*, (2014) 25(1):1–18.

21 Cox, LM and Blaser, MJ 'Antibiotics in Early Life and Obesity.' *Nature Reviews Endocrinology*, (2015) 11(3):182–190.

22 Clapp, M et al. 'Gut Microbiota's Effect on Mental Health: The Gut-Brain Axis.' *Clinical Practice*, (2017) 7(4):987.

23 'Microbes Help Produce Serotonin in Gut.' California Institute of Technology, (2015). Retrieved from http://www.caltech.edu/

24 Rea K et al. 'The Microbiome: A Key Regulator of Stress and Neuroinflammation.' *Neurobiology of Stress*, (2016) 4:23-33.

25 Galland, L 'The Gut Microbiome and the Brain.' *Journal of Medicinal Food*, (2014) 17(12):1261–1272.

26 Selhub EM et al. 'Fermented Foods, Microbiota, and Mental Health: Ancient Practice Meets Nutritional Psychiatry.' *Journal of Physiological Anthropology*, (2014) 33(1):2.

27 Newman, T 'How Inflammation and Gut Bacteria Influence Autism.' *Medical News Today*, (2018). Retrieved from http://www.medicalnewstoday.com/

28 Peterson, M 'Emerging Evidence Behind the Gut-Skin Axis Theory.' *BioCeuticals*, (2016). Retrieved from http://www.bioceuticals.com.au/

29 Al Roujayee A 'Cutaneous Manifestations of Inflammatory Bowel Disease.' *Saudi Journal of Gastroenterology*, (2007) 13:159-62.

30 Slominski, A 'A Nervous Breakdown in the Skin: Stress and the Epidermal Barrier.' *Journal of Clinical Investigation*, (2007) 117(11):3166–3169.

31 Bowe WP and Logan AC 'Acne Vulgaris, Probiotics and the Gut-Brain-Skin Axis – Back to the Future?' *Gut Pathogens*, (2011) 3(1):1.

32 Weiss, E and Rajani, K 'Diet and Rosacea: The Role of Dietary Change in the Management of Rosacea.' *Dermatology Practical & Conceptual*, (2017) 7(4):31–37.

33 Forno, E et al. 'Diversity of the Gut Microbiota and Eczema in Early Life.' *Clinical and Molecular Allergy*, (2008) 6:11.

34 Mosca, A et al. 'Gut Microbiota Diversity and Human Diseases: Should We Reintroduce Key Predators in Our Ecosystem?' *Frontiers in Microbiology*, (2016) 7:455.

35 Gruber R et al. 'Sebaceous Gland, Hair Shaft, and Epidermal Barrier Abnormalities in Keratosis Pilaris With and Without Filaggrin Deficiency.' *American Journal of Pathology*, (2015) 185(4):1012-21.

36 Fasano, A 'Zonulin, Regulation of Tight Junctions, and Autoimmune Diseases.' *Annals of the New York Academy of Sciences*, (2012) 1258(1):25–33.

37 Altobelli, E et al. 'Low-FODMAP Diet Improves Irritable Bowel Syndrome Symptoms: A Meta-Analysis.' *Nutrients*, (2017) 9(9).

38 Marco, ML et al. 'Health Benefits of Fermented Foods: Microbiota and Beyond.' *Current Opinion in Biotechnology*, (2017) 44:94–102.

39 Tzounis, X et al. 'Prebiotic Evaluation of Cocoa-Derived Flavanols in Healthy Humans by Using a Randomized, Controlled, Double-Blind, Crossover Intervention Study.' *American Journal of Clinical Nutrition*, (2011) 93(1):62–72.

40 Flint, HJ et al. 'Microbial Degradation of Complex Carbohydrates in the Gut.' *Gut Microbes*, (2012) 3(4):289–306.

41 Courage, KH 'Fiber-Famished Gut Microbes Linked to Poor Health.' *Scientific American*, (2015). Retrieved from http://www.scientificamerican.com/

42 Holscher, HD 'Dietary Fiber and Prebiotics and the Gastrointestinal Microbiota.' *Gut Microbes*, (2017) 8(2):172–184.

43 Birt, DF et al. 'Resistant Starch: Promise for Improving Human Health.' *Advances in Nutrition*, (2013) 4(6):587–601.

44 University of Wisconsin-Madison. 'Study Reveals Gene Expression Changes with Meditation.' *ScienceDaily*, (2013). Retrieved from http://www.sciencedaily.com/

45 Deaver JA et al. 'Circadian Disruption Changes Gut Microbiome Taxa and Functional Gene Composition.' *Frontiers in Microbiology*, (2018) 9:737.

46 Scudellari, M 'News Feature: Cleaning Up the Hygiene Hypothesis.' *Proceedings of the National Academy of Sciences of the United States of America*, (2017) 114(7):1433–1436.

47 Whiteman, H 'Exercise Alone Alters Our Gut Microbiota.' *Medical News Today*, (2017). Retrieved from http://www.medicalnewstoday.com/

48 Smits, SA et al. 'Seasonal Cycling in the Gut Microbiome Of The Hadza Hunter-Gatherers Of Tanzania.' *Science*, (2017) 357(6353):802–806.

49 Shen, R et al. 'Role of a Brain–Gut Axis in Energy Balance.' *Proceedings of the National Academy of Sciences*, (2016) 113(23):E3307-E3314.

Index

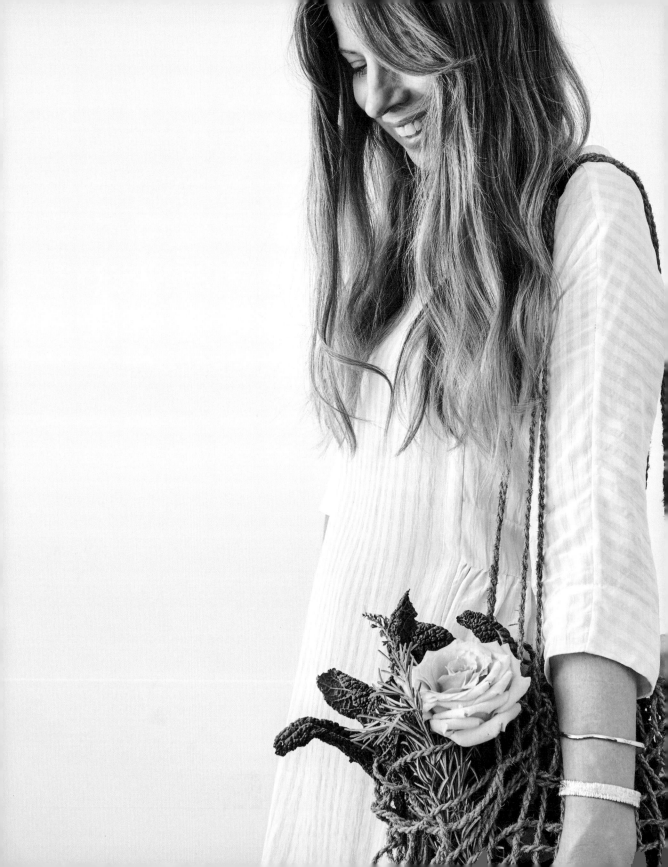

Acknowledgements

It takes a community of microbes for good gut health and a community of great people to make a book. I'd like to thank Dr Andrew Holmes at The Charles Perkins Centre, Sydney University, and naturopath Alison Cassar for your wonderful guidance and support while writing this book, as well as nutritionist Georgia Bellas and naturopath Rhiona Robertson for all your help and input. I am very grateful.

Thanks so much to Ashley Cameron for your contribution to the content, Michala Johnston for your second set of eyes, and Rachael Lane – for your dedication. I love working on recipes with you and really appreciate all the late nights and hours and hours of discussion (about flavour and FODMAP). Thanks also to the Beauty Chef team and my lovely EA Larissa Morozoff. And of course, thank you to Lee Blaylock and Rochelle Eagle and Evi O: what an awesome creative team!

Last but not least, thank you to my editor Kate Armstrong, and Anna Collett and Jane Willson for all your wonderful support at Hardie Grant.

This edition published in 2024 by Hardie Grant Books,
an imprint of Hardie Grant Publishing
First published in 2019

Hardie Grant Books (Melbourne)
Building 1, 658 Church Street
Richmond, Victoria 3121

Hardie Grant North America
2912 Telegraph Ave
Berkeley, California 94705

hardiegrant.com/books

Hardie Grant acknowledges the Traditional Owners of the
Country on which we work, the Wurundjeri People of the
Kulin Nation and the Gadigal People of the Eora Nation,
and recognises their continuing connection to the land,
waters and culture. We pay our respects to their Elders past
and present.

A catalogue record for this
book is available from the
National Library of Australia

The Beauty Chef Gut Guide
ISBN 978 1 76145 115 7

10 9 8 7 6 5 4 3 2 1

Publisher: Simon Davis
Head of Editorial: Jasmin Chua
Editor: Kate J Armstrong
Design Manager: Kristin Thomas
Cover Designer: Daniel New
Designer: Evi-O.Studio
Photographer: Rochelle Eagle
Stylist: Lee Blaylock
Recipe Developer: Rachael Lane
Head of Production: Todd Rechner
Production Controller: Jessica Harvie
Dress by Lee Mathews
Jewellery by Lucy Folk

Colour reproduction by Splitting Image Colour Studio
Printed in China by Leo Paper Products. LTD

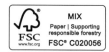

MIX
Paper | Supporting
responsible forestry
FSC® C020056

The paper this book is printed on is from FSC®-certified
forests and other sources. FSC® promotes environmentally
responsible, socially beneficial and economically viable
management of the world's forests.